SPIRITUALLY FIT

A Fitness Program You Can Have Faith In
by Clark Bartram

CB Enterprises
Escondido, CA

Notice

Before beginning any exercise program, consult your physician. The author and publisher disclaim any liability, personal or professional, resulting from the application or misapplication of any of the information in this publication.

Library of Congress Cataloging-in-Publication Data

Xxxxx Xxxxx Xx

Printed in the United States of America

Please order additional copies at www.clarkbartram.com.

SPIRITUALLY FIT is available for bulk purchase, special promotions, and premiums. Please email inquiries to: clark@clarkbartram.com

Book Design: David Sparks

Cover Photography: Garrett Thomas

Additional Photos: Jason Ellis

Lord I thank you for my body and the ability to be active and healthy. I ask that you give me balance as I move forward with my exercise and nutritional program. I pray Lord that you give me the ability to remain focused and avoid and any temptation that I may encounter while in the gym atmosphere. I will not covet anyone else's body nor will I become envious of anyone I meet.

I choose to love myself as I am and will be a positive example to my children, friends and all I come into contact with on a daily basis.

I thank you Lord that I am becoming more and more Spiritually Fit each day.

This book is dedicated to all people who desire to achieve a healthy balance in life and who are interested in using their God-given gifts to inspire others.

You can do it!

"The man who does not read good books has no advantage over the man who cannot read them."

-- Mark Twain

Fitness and faith — where is the balance? How do we as Christians justify spending time trying to develop our bodies when we know that the body is temporary and superficial? Is it right to be concerned with how we look? How does God feel about it? How do we achieve the proper equilibrium between our physical and spiritual selves?

These are all valid questions, but they can also be the basis for lame excuses. I've seen many people rationalize their way out of exercise and eating right because they think, or want to think, that God wouldn't approve.

My hope is that this book will help you understand that we as Christians should put our best foot forward in all areas of life, including our physical health and appearance.

I give you all the tools you need to develop your best body and use it to enrich your faith and get the most out of life.

This project is the result of the constant flow of comments and questions I get about how my very public fitness lifestyle relates to me as a Christian. Throughout the entire Christian community, I've noticed that many people are genuinely interested in becoming Spiritually Fit.

Blessings,
Clark Bartram

Contents

Chapter One

How God Sent The Power Team To Change My Life

"We never become truly spiritual by sitting down and wishing to become so. You must undertake something so great that you cannot accomplish it unaided."

-- Phillips Brooks

As a professional fitness model devoted to God, I've had to work hard to find the right balance between my physical side and my spiritual side. I found God relatively late in life, and walking with Him has given me even more motivation to stay fit and healthy for myself, my family, my community, and my Creator. This is my personal story of how God entered my life.

I Was Just Minding My Own Business!

I was saved in 1988 at a Power Team meeting in Escondido, California. My salvation came after a young man approached me at the gym I managed. I was giving my typical sales speech when I came to my famous go-for-the-money line. I said to the guy, "You know, procrastination is health's number-one enemy. You need to get this membership today."

Much to my surprise, this bold young man turned the tables on me like no other person had done in my life of 25 years. His reply was, "You know, procrastination could be your number-one enemy if you don't get your life right with God!"

Who did this nerd think he was? How could a skinny goof like him say something like that to me? Didn't he know who I was? Couldn't he see my 230-pound, muscular body? Didn't he see the bodybuilding trophies in my office?

"Man, I'm not interested in that God stuff," was my reply.

He didn't buy a membership, and I didn't buy into God that day, either. As far as I was concerned, if the best God could do was send me some skinny little kid, He didn't really know anything about me at all.

Something did happen, though. That skinny Christian goofball got under my skin. He didn't see all of my physical attributes, but he saw the emptiness that I thought was well hidden under my facade of finely tuned muscle. I got on my knees that night and asked God, if He was real, to send me someone I could relate to, in a physical sense, to lead me on the path to His grace.

One week later, I was sitting at the front desk of the gym when a lady walked in with a poster. "Can I hang this on your wall?" she asked, very politely. "Yeah, anywhere you want," I smiled. She chose the wall directly in front of me and unrolled the colorful poster. The poster featured six bodybuilders — all much bigger than me, I might add! It proclaimed that "God Made You To Win." My heart began to race. I was beginning to fear, hope, and wonder if God really had heard my prayer. About two hours later, it became obvious to me that God had indeed heard my call for help when I met Mike Hagen, a member of the Power Team.

This guy could have been my big brother — we looked that much alike. The only difference was that he was about 20-30 pounds heavier and more muscular than I was! This was beginning to get weird! He introduced himself, casually mentioned the Power Team, and proceeded to get his workout in. I sat at my desk, spinning with emotion and expectation.

After 20 minutes of talking to myself about what was actually going on, I made my way over to where Mike was training. We talked about working out, football, and other guy stuff. When I found out that he had been a professional football player, my heart really began to race. Not because I was meeting some star, but because playing pro ball was a dream of mine as a child.

I grew up in Canton, Ohio, home of the Pro Football Hall of Fame. Every kid in Canton lived for football. I played in hundreds of Super Bowls and was always the hero of the game, scoring on the last drive when time was running out. These Super Bowls were in the field next to my house, and my heroics were in my imagination as I ran across the field that seemed so big as a child.

It was at this point in my conversation with Mike that I was beginning to realize that maybe I could have a relationship with God and still find room for physical fitness. I felt somewhat comfortable telling Mike what I was going through in my life.

I was on the verge of a break-up with a girl named Anita, who I cared about deeply. I loved her, but I didn't want to admit it. I would break up with her when it was good for me, and then get back together with her when I felt I was at risk of losing her. I felt bad on occasion, but was unable to deal with my issues. She was getting smart, and was finally ready to give me the boot — deservedly so.

For a brief moment, I opened up and let someone I didn't know into my hidden place of vulnerability and insecurity. He immediately seized the opportunity by racking his 80-pound dumbbells and hugging me. I began to cry, right in the middle of the gym, and felt a sense of love that I hadn't felt in a long time. Mike and I talked some more, and he invited me to the Power Team meeting that night.

As soon as he left, however, the devil began to steal the seed that was planted. I began to feel embarrassed, and doubted that all this was some master plan designed by God to help me. God couldn't really know me that well or care about me that much. Nah, it couldn't be happening.

I called my girlfriend Anita and told her about what happened. She listened to me with love and understanding that I didn't deserve from her, and encouraged me to attend the meeting. She even offered to come along.

When it was time to leave for the meeting, I didn't want anyone at work to think I was going to some crazy religious event. So I took the lead box and told everyone that I was going to the meeting to get some prospects for the health club. That was my excuse, while I secretly hoped that this thing was for real.

Anita and I arrived at the meeting and were escorted to the front row where seats had been reserved for me. "I like this VIP treatment," I thought to myself! I was seated next to the host Pastor who invited the Power Team to our town. Out of respect for him, I asked Anita not to throw her leg over mine while we were seated. I wasn't a completely terrible guy!

I felt the excitement build as music started to play, and the crowd rose as the Power Team was introduced. "Weighing in at 275 pounds, able to bench press 500 pounds, please welcome Barry Handly!..." The introductions continued, and I was impressed with each one. I was a champion bodybuilder who just recently called God to the carpet, and He was teaching me a lesson.

I watched in amazement as the team members blew up hot water bottles till they exploded, broke baseball bats with their bare hands, and smashed through mountains of ice and brick. By now, I was clapping and jumping like one of the little kids in the crowd! I was completely drawn into the world of the Power Team, which was really my world. It was what I knew, loved, and related to.

When the excitement of the show died down, I told Anita that I was ready to leave. I didn't want to sit through some preaching thing for the next hour. But suddenly, Mike came up with a microphone and began to share his story to the crowd. At first, I thought he was telling my story! Who had given him the scoop about what I had dealt with as a child? Who told him about my divorced parents, and the stress that caused in my life?

Again, the similarities between Mike and me were spooky, and when I realized he hadn't spied into my life, my heart began to race with anticipation about what would happen next. Maybe God really did know me after all, and maybe these guys were sent just for me. I felt something big happening and wanted to jump from my seat.

After Mike finished his testimony, John Jacobs, the lead member of the Power Team, continued to wear down my defenses. "Many of you think that just because you're nice and never hurt anyone you will earn your way into heaven," he said. "Some of you think you can make it to heaven on your good deeds." Well, this was me and he shot my theory down when he quoted John 3:3 — "You must first be born again to enter the kingdom of heaven!"

After he said this, he invited the crowd to come forward for this salvation thing I kept hearing about. The next thing I remember, I was standing at the altar surrounded by hundreds of others, listening to this guy pray that God would forgive our sins. How did I end up down here? Why was I crying? Why did all this feel so good to me? By this time, I was realizing that the boldness of that skinny kid was really paying off — and he didn't even have a clue about the impact his words were having at that very moment.

In the midst of my emotion, I was given another obvious sign that God did know me and sent these guys just for me. I was standing there basking in the joy of the moment when John Jacobs pointed to me and called me to come up on stage by saying, "Young man, God has a plan for your life!" I looked behind me for the young man he was pointing to, and he said it again with more emphasis. "You, in the pink shirt, God wants to use you to do great things!"

Oh boy, he was talking to me! What do I do now? I didn't have much time to think when he called me to come join him on stage. I stood there surrounded by six guys, all bigger and stronger than me, as they prayed for God to work in my life. I thought I had cried in the gym, but it was nothing compared to the tears, snot, and everything else that shamelessly came streaming out of my face. It felt good. I felt release. I knew at this moment that God loved me enough to send a group of bodybuilding preachers to save me. But what next?

I sat with the guys for a while and we talked about many things, mainly about how I should act upon my newfound life of serving God. How was I supposed to do it? These guys were flying out in a few days. Who would I relate to then, and how would I continue to learn?

I had no clue, but they did. John Jacobs told me, "Go to work tomorrow, quit your job, go to this church three times a week, and work out hard. We're going to come back for you in a few months."

"How will I pay my bills?" I thought to myself.

But before I could get the words out John said, "Don't worry about money. We'll take care of everything for you."

What a night! All my sins were forgiven, I no longer had to work, all my bills were going to be paid by someone else, and I got to work out all the time!

I went to work the next day with an empty lead box and a full heart, ready to start my new life. I walked into owner's office and gave him the news. "I quit." One of the other people in the room joked, "What, did you get saved at that meeting last night or something?"

"Yes I did," was my serious reply.

I cleaned out my desk and didn't look back. I attended church every time the doors were opened and I worked out like a man on a mission. Anita, who was also saved at the Power Team meeting, and I began to put the pieces of our strained relationship back together. I began to respect and consider her feelings. I tried to be what I was learning a man should be. We grew together and things began looking better.

I was at a friend's house when the phone rang. It was John Jacobs from the Power Team. "Hey, we want to take you on the road now," he said. Wow, he actually did what he said he was going to do! That was new to me. But how did he find me at my friend's house? And how was I going to tell Anita that I was leaving?

We worked it all out and I went on the road with the Power Team. I did whatever they asked me to do to serve. I carried bags, folded t-shirts, mailed posters, and cleaned bathrooms. You name it I did it, and I was happy to do so. I was learning and growing, realizing that there was a whole other world out there, a world of encouraging people who helped others instead of hurting them. A world of giving, not just taking. I liked it and felt that maybe God did have a plan for me.

After serving for a year and a half, I had hoped that I would get to do stunts and be "on the team" in a more formal sense. Well, I found out the hard way that this wasn't a part of God's plan for my life. I was very depressed and let down.

But in hindsight, I realized that God knows best and that His plans are bigger and better than ours. Even though I never had the chance to rip one phone book, blow up one hot water bottle, or break a stack of concrete, the whole experience was one of the best things that ever happened to me, because God came into my life and has never left me. God used the Power Team to reach me when no one else could, and because of that I am blessed.

I went on to marry Anita. We now have two wonderful children, Taylor and Mitch, and I'm living God's purpose for my life.

My goal in this book is to help you live a healthier, happier life through an appreciation of your physical self, and to show you the many parallels between the spiritual and the physical. I want to help you understand that God wants you to achieve your best body, so you can better serve Him and enjoy His many blessings.

Chapter Two

You're Not Who You Are Because Of Your Body

"You need to learn to be happy by nature, because you'll seldom have the chance to be happy by circumstance."

-- Lavetta Sue Wegman

It's no secret that the reverence of physical beauty is way out of proportion in our culture today. Everywhere you look — in magazines and catalogs, on television, and in the movies — sex sells. Now, I don't think it's inherently bad to appreciate human beauty, but in recent years our obsession with the body has made multi-millionaires out of supermodels, created a huge demand for breast implants and other surgical procedures, and otherwise put pressure on people in our society to meet the media's current idea of the physical ideal.

Even though I'm a paid, professional fitness model, I believe that our society puts too much emphasis on the body as the definition of who we are as people. I've heard countless people tell me things like, "If I could only lose ten pounds, then I'd be happy." Or, "If only my breasts were bigger, I'd be more confident." Believe me, I've met people who appear to have it all, and yet they're still unhappy. And I've seen people continually reach their goals, only to put off their happiness till they reach the next thing they think will make them happy.

The worst comment I get is when people tell me, "If only I had a body like yours..." This makes me cringe because I got into the fitness business to help people become the best they can be, not to wish they were like me. I want to inspire people to make better lifestyle choices, not to feel bad about themselves because they're not on the cover of a magazine.

I work hard at what I do, and it's taken a great deal of persistence, a pleasant attitude, a fierce commitment, and impeccable integrity to reach the level of success I've achieved. There's a lot more to being a fitness model than just being in shape and showing up for photo shoots! And as for the physical part, I make no bones about the fact that genetics has played a big role in my physical development. Although I train very hard and eat perfectly most of the time, it's really God who has blessed me with the genetics to succeed in my chosen line of work and in my ministry.

I've met a lot of people during my career, and I've often wondered why some people are motivated by the media's suggestion of perfection while others use media images to diminish their self-esteem. I've often wondered why some people strive to "live the lifestyle," while others think the models in the magazines are sinful or unholy. And I've often wondered why some people are inspired by physical beauty while others just get jealous.

My belief is that when the spirit is weak we give more importance to the illusion of the body. We tend to look on the outside for fulfillment rather than on the inside, and we tend to criticize things we think are threatening to us, and open ourselves to the sin of jealousy.

We all know that jealousy is a sin (Gal 5:20), mentioned along with antagonism, rivalry, bad temper, quarrels, disagreements, factions, and malice. In a physical world, it's only natural to compare ourselves with others, even though we know deep down that all of us are equal in the eyes of God.

Comparison turns into the sin of jealousy when we use the observation of our differences to destroy the feelings of joy and peace we should feel as creatures uniquely made and loved by God. On the other hand, comparing ourselves to others can inspire us to do better in the physical world, as long as we're able to see the big picture that goes beyond the limits of the body and embraces the eternal realm of the spirit.

This idea that we need a balance between our physical and spiritual selves became real to me after a conversation with my dear friend James DeMelo, a bodybuilder turned evangelist. He said he was praying one day about his bodybuilding competitions and how they related to his walk with God. Was it right for him to compete against other men to see who had the best body? Did God approve of this seemingly superficial activity?

As James prayed, God showed him images of the physical James and the spiritual James. What he saw shocked him. His physical self was strong and muscular, while the spiritual James was weak and looked as if he were starving. It was then that he realized he needed balance. It wasn't that God wanted him to stop training, or even competing. He wanted James to find a balance that would raise his spirit.

God wants that for all of us. He wants us to focus as much, or more, on our spirits as we do on our bodies, but not at the expense of the physical. If we're unhealthy and lacking energy, how will we be able to do good in a hurting world?

For all of us, the body is a temporary thing. Whether you have great genetics or struggle with diseases or disabilities that are out of your control, the body does not endure. But while the body has limitations, our spirits do not. Your spirit has an unlimited capacity for love, kindness, generosity, and forgiveness. The sin isn't that we take care of our bodies or even take pleasure in our physicality, it's that we worship the physical over the spiritual when they're both important players in our human experience.

You're not who you are because of your body, but you are who you are because of your spirit. And when that spirit is bolstered by a healthy, nourished, and active body, I believe that you're better able to experience joy in life and better able to fulfill your responsibilities as a Christian.

Chapter Three

Your Body Can Unleash Your Spirit

"Things do not change; we change."
-- Henry David Thoreau

I'll never forget the day I got saved. Of course, it was a wonderful, life-changing experience, but something else happened that day which remains indelibly printed in my mind.

It was a simple comment that came from a young Christian man who was probably fairly new to the faith, as well. Just moments after I had accepted Jesus into my heart and was still weeping from the weight of sin that had been lifted from me, this guy approached me and said, "Are you going to stop working out now?" The subtext of the question was, "you can stop wasting your time working on your body, because your soul has just been taken care of for eternity."

This struck me as an odd comment, given the whole context of the Power Team's very physical ministry. I can distinctly remember the look of disgust on this kid's face as he expressed his opinion that my chosen profession was an absolute abomination to God. Maybe a drug dealer or a mafia boss would have a hard time justifying his employment decision as a Christian, but a fitness professional?

His comment shook me a little bit since everything was happening so fast, and I did question how I could balance my newfound faith with the physical pursuits I loved so much. Did I really have to give up the things in life that fulfilled me to be a good Christian? Were my efforts to build my body going to stunt my spiritual growth?

It didn't take me long to figure out that the kid who made the comment was either really excited or had some really bad experience in the gym! But I'm glad that he told me how he felt, because it caused me to really see how a healthy, fit body can do wonders for the soul.

First of all, I realized that my life-long commitment to physical exercise gave me the discipline I needed to go to Church, study the Bible, and become a role model in my spiritual community. You read in my testimony how I quit my job at the gym, went to Church every time the doors were open, and worked out hard until I traveled with the Power Team. I could never have done that without my years of physical training.

Furthermore, my early experiences with the Power Team helped me decide to use fitness as my ministry. My God-given body helped me become a devoted Christian, and I believed that I could help others find God through physical well-being.

As I pursued this goal, I went through many phases. There were times when all I did was "preach" to people. It even got to the point where my family didn't want to hear from me anymore, because I was so obnoxious and didn't show any sensitivity! I had to learn some hard lessons and refine my approach. As I grew, I continued to see strong parallels between physical health and spiritual well-being in my dealings with personal training clients, friends, fans, and members of my congregation.

I saw how fit people tended to have more zest for life than their out-of-shape counterparts. I saw how people with energy were more open to trying new things, helping others, and getting the most out of life. I saw how healthy people were more engaged in the world. And personally, I know when I'm feeling fit, healthy, and full of energy, I feel like I can accomplish anything!

It dawned on me that if more Christians could understand the power of physical fitness, the more effective we could be as a community. If more Christians could exercise and eat right, the more their spirits could open up to joyful experience.

We all know that the Bible says your body is a temple of the Holy Spirit. Now, I've heard that scripture explained a few different ways, but no matter what your interpretation of it is I think we can all agree that the human body is a gift from God. And if we as Christians believe this, then why do so many of us accept being unhealthy and ineffective in life and in our ministries because we don't have the energy?

Personally, I think the argument that our bodies are only temporary and that it's the soul that needs our attention for eternal happiness is a cop out. It's true, our physical being doesn't endure, but I don't think that's a good excuse to avoid taking care of yourself while you're on earth. God gave you your body for the purpose of exploring the human condition in all its dimensions — mental, physical, and spiritual — and by taking care of your body you can attend to the soul in extremely rich and beneficial ways.

The key is to find your personal balance, so that your body nurtures your soul and your spirituality nurtures your body. Approach your body with reverence and be grateful to God for it. Find joy in physical exercise and movement. When your motivation is pure, there's no reason to feel guilty or shameful about your body. And when you understand that the benefits of a healthier body are greater than yourself, you can actually celebrate the time you take to care for your body in the gym, at the dinner table, or walking around the block.

What's more, you'll be better able to deal with a healthy, fit body when you're grounded spiritually. Find your balance now, so when you do reach your goals you won't freak out, divorce your spouse, and throw it all back in the face of God and everyone who supported you along the way!

The moral of this chapter is that you're the steward of the body God gave you, and that you can use your body as a tool for God's service. By respecting your body and treating it right, you can be more effective in your ministry and be a better role model in the Christian community.

So what are you waiting for? Unleash your body...it will unleash your spirit!

Chapter Four

Your Body And
The Power Of Belief

*"Nothing can stop the man with the right mental attitude
from achieving his goal; nothing on earth can help the
man with the wrong mental attitude."*
--Thomas Jefferson

It seems the minute you say words like "meditate," "affirmations,"
or "positive thinking," many Christians back away or get offended.
There's a pervasive belief in the Christian community that metaphysical or "New Age" concepts "aren't from the Lord."
But getting caught up in our own vernacular can limit us when it
comes to developing lifestyle patterns conducive to good health and
fitness. I'm not suggesting that anyone compromise his or her
beliefs, and I'm not a follower of the New Age movement, but I do
think it's important to be less judgmental and more open minded.
You may be surprised to discover that many "New Age" concepts
are really age-old truths that are discussed throughout the Bible
itself. If you look in the Book of Psalms, for example, the word
"Selah" is used over and over again. It means to meditate on what
you just read. Ephesians 4:23 offers the opportunity "to be made
new in the attitude of your minds." And Romans 12:2 proclaims, "be
ye transformed by the renewing of your mind."
I could go on and on with examples proving that God wants you to
think positively, have a great attitude, and live to your fullest poten-
tial, but that really isn't my job. My goal in this chapter is to give you
some tried and true mental exercises that, when done in the spirit of
love and faith, will inspire you to reach the fitness goals you set for
yourself.
As these exercises become second nature to you through practice
and repetition, you'll get a bonus — you can use them to enrich
your other daily habits as a man or woman of God, such as praying,
getting the most out of your weekly service, and relating to others.
Robert MacPhee Helped Me See The Light
I was holding a fitness seminar for 100 participants when a man by
the name of Robert MacPhee asked if he could address my group on

the subject of the mental aspect of their fitness regimen. I must admit that I was one of those reluctant, over-zealous Christians at the time, and I feared that his message would infect the minds of my students with metaphysical garbage!

I tried to listen to him with an open mind, however, and after reviewing his material I realized that Biblical principles were the foundation of his message. If you really think about it, nearly every motivational speaker uses principles directly from the Bible, without always giving credit where credit is due.

So I let Robert address my group, and as he spoke I could see that his message resonated with many of the seminar participants. He talked about how people tend to sabotage success by subconsciously reliving past failures. When it comes to fitness, we set ourselves up for disappointment with beliefs like "Diets never work for me;" "I can't ever seem to gain any muscle;" or "I'm destined to be fat because my whole family is fat."

Out With The Negative, In With The Positive

Our thought patterns have a powerful impact on what we achieve in life, but we don't have to be stuck in negative patterns. Just like many of us have come to our faith later in life, we can re-train our minds to believe positive thoughts at any point on our journey. According to my friend Robert MacPhee, changing what you hold true in your mind will help you stop the cycle of self-doubt and thoughts of failure so you can become who you really want to be, regardless of past failures or family history. Through positive "self talk," you can create a new self-image that can lead you to positive results and healthier beliefs about your place in humanity. As the Bible says, (Proverbs 23:7 [NAS]) "As he thinks within himself so he is."

This is how it works. Self talk (our thoughts) directly affects our self-image (our beliefs), and our beliefs affect our thoughts. If we believe we don't have time to exercise, for example, we'll think the thoughts of a person who doesn't have time to exercise, and that just strengthens our beliefs. It can be a self-perpetuating cycle that keeps us stuck in bad patterns of behavior. Robert MacPhee, in his Heart Set on Fitness program, points out that we have the power to choose whether to accept our current self-image or create a new one.

OUR THOUGHTS AND BELIEFS ARE DIRECTLY CONNECTED

THOUGHTS

↑ ↓

SELF-IMAGE (BELIEFS)

By changing our self-image, it becomes easier to take direct action and make other changes in our lives. Actions are the physical steps we take to bring about expected results. They're caused by external influences that suggest we should be making some changes.

RESULTS FOLLOW ACTIONS

EXTERNAL ACTIONS ──────→ INFLUENCE RESULTS

When our self-image matches the results we're looking for, our actions can be extremely powerful. But when our self-image is out of sync with the results we want, change becomes difficult, if not impossible. That's why it's important to work on our thoughts and self-image before, or at least at the same time as, we take direct action.

ACTIONS ARE MORE EFFECTIVE WHEN THE RESULTS WE WANT ARE IN LINE WITH OUR BELIEFS

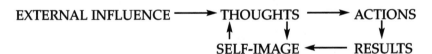

EXTERNAL INFLUENCE ──→ THOUGHTS ──→ ACTIONS

↑ ↓ ↓

SELF-IMAGE ←── RESULTS

Affirming Your Goals

The first thing you need to do is decide what you want to achieve. Do you want bigger muscles or a slimmer waist? Do you want to eat better? Do you want to be a more loving wife or husband? Write everything down.

When you have your list of goals in front of you, the next thing you do is select the two or three that are most important to you. Write down an affirmation for each of these goals. An affirmation is a simple statement that creates a vivid picture of a goal in your mind, as if it has already been achieved.

Your affirmations should be as specific as possible, and should be in the present, not the future, tense. Robert suggests that each one of your affirmations meet these five criteria:

1. Starts with "I am"
2. Is short and specific
3. Is positive (the mind doesn't respond to words like don't, not, no, etc.)
4. Includes an action word ending in "ing"
5. Includes a feeling word (how will you feel when you've reached your goal?)

Here are some examples of affirmations as they relate to people who want to be spiritually fit:

- I am 130 pounds and am excited to be wearing a size 6 dress!
- I am energetic from eating only fresh, whole foods to nourish my body.
- I am proudly completing my daily gym workout.
- I am calmly and contemplatively reading one chapter of the Bible each day.
- I experience love and practice forgiveness while I am relating to others.

Keep your list of affirmations with you at all times and say each affirmation OUT LOUD as many times a day as you can to help your mind believe in your new reality. As you say each affirmation OUT LOUD, create a corresponding visual picture in your mind. See yourself as healthy, fit, attractive, and loving. See yourself with bigger muscles or a slimmer waist. See yourself making smart nutrition choices. And always remember to consider how the accomplishment of your specific goals will make you feel. This affirmation exercise is probably the most important thing you can do if you're serious about reaching your goals.

Putting Your Goals In The Context Of Your Life

At this point, some of you are probably thinking that this is pretty silly stuff. But I promise you, it works! Robert MacPhee has a good way to motivate you to keep going with your affirmations.

Every day, think about the association between your goals and the things that are most important in your life. Think of how much better your relationships with your spouse, your kids, your parents, your friends, your co-workers, your congregation, and even God Himself will be as you progress toward your goals.

One way to get clear on these associations is to repeatedly ask yourself probing questions to define and justify your goals. Questions like "What do I want?", "Why is that important to me?", and "What will this get me?" can all help you identify what really is important to you.

By always keeping an eye on the richness that will enter your life as you achieve your goals (which is especially true with health and fitness because it impacts every other area of our lives), you'll be motivated to keep saying your affirmations no matter what you currently think about them.

Putting What The Mind Thinks Into Motion

The last exercise in our little mental trinity of thoughts, beliefs, and actions is to continually ask yourself what Robert MacPhee calls the bridge question. It's a question that bridges the gap between the image you have in your mind about who you want to be and the behavior you must put into action to reach your goals.

The bridge question is simply "What would a (type of person I want to be) person be DOING today?" This would be my personal example of a bridge question: What would a spiritually balanced, physically fit, healthy, God-loving person be doing today? Would he or she be watching television or going to the gym for an invigorating workout? Would he or she be stressing out over a family matter, or trying to resolve the problem by open communication? Would he or she be going to McDonald's? Would he or she be having a soda or a glass of water? You get the idea.

Try it with everything you do. Ask yourself if the person you want to be would be doing what you're doing right now. The person you want to be would definitely be reading this book, so you're already off to a great start!

Persistence Pays Off

As you do these exercises, you're going to encounter resistance. You might doubt the power of these exercises and think they won't work. Those around you may think what you're doing is stupid or remind you of your past failures.

Try to be persistent even in the face of negative thinking. It took you years to develop negative thought patterns, so it's going to take some time to replace them with positive ones.

Throughout this book, I constantly remind you that you're not perfect, and I don't mean that as a criticism. I only say it so that small setbacks don't discourage you and lead to bigger failures. If you expect and accept setbacks, and know that God is with you every step of the way, you'll be less likely to give up completely. Try and be forgiving, learn from your mistakes, and stay focused on your goals. They do come from God, and they're worth working toward.

Robert MacPhee's Top Three Mind Exercises For Health and Happiness.

1. Repeat affirmations several times per day. This is probably the most important thing you can do to improve your life. (Remember Ephesians 4:23, "be made new in the attitude of your minds.")

2. Remind yourself each day of the association between health and fitness and the things that are most important in your life. You'll be more motivated when you think about how achieving your goals will help you relate to your family, per form at your job, and be a model Christian.

3. Keep asking yourself the "bridge question." This gets you from image to action by asking "What would a (type of person I want to be) person be DOING today?"

To learn more about Robert MacPhee, visit his Web site at www.heartset.com.

Chapter Five

Going To The Gym
Is Like Going To Church

*"As long as I see any thing to be done for God, life is worth having;
but O how vain and unworthy it is to live for any lower end!"*
-- David Brainerd

All of us go to church regularly to strengthen our faith. By going to
hear the Word of God each week, we reinforce His message of Love
for an imperfect world. Think about how you feel after a service —
chances are you leave the building feeling excited, energized, and
more connected to God

Well, the same thing happens when you exercise regularly. You
strengthen your body with each workout, and chances are you'll
leave the gym feeling excited, energized, and even more connected
to God!

It takes the same type of discipline to go to the gym as it does to go
to Church, so if you can do one you can certainly do the other. And
both offer rewards that far outweigh the hassles of leaving the
house for an hour!

In this chapter, I'm going to give you all the tools you need to get
results at the gym, or even at your own house if you have the equipment. Think of it like the church bulletin that guides you through
the service.

Stick With The Basics

In all my years of helping people achieve better health and fitness,
I've discovered that when you start with the basics and stick with
the basics, you're going to achieve results.

Just as we Christians practice basic activities to improve our spiritual health — like prayer, fellowship, and Bible study — there are certain things we must do in order to get the most out of an exercise
program.

We can look at prayer, for example, as exercise for the spirit. Praying
consistently will strengthen your relationship with the Lord, just like
exercising consistently will help you sculpt your body, burn fat, and
improve the health of your heart.

Reading the Bible gives us a rest from our daily cares, and prepares us for making the right choices in a stressful world. With physical training, the rest we take between exercise sessions prepares us for the stresses of the next workout and helps our bodies respond to training in a positive way.

And fellowship with other believers can be likened to proper nutrition. Really living our faith with others nourishes the spirit, just as eating the right nutrients nourishes the body.

If you can follow these guidelines, you'll get good results no matter what your position is in life, and no matter what exercise routine you follow. There are a lot of different training programs out there, a multitude of exercise gadgets to choose from, and a variety of philosophies about when and how to exercise. But don't sweat the details — I've found that no one program is inherently better than another.

What works for you may not work for someone else. There are lots of factors involved, including what you enjoy doing, what you can fit in your schedule, and what training facilities are available.

Here's an example of what I mean. My personal preference is to do aerobic training AFTER I lift weights. This has worked well for me over the years, but I'm not going to sit here and say that you won't get in shape if you do aerobic training before you lift weights, or even on alternate days. Some people say that you should do your aerobic training at 5:00 a.m. This is limiting, because when you think you have to do it at 5:00 a.m. and you can't do it at 5:00 a.m., then you might not do it all. Or you might do it some other time and feel guilty that you're not doing it at 5:00 a.m.! That's no way to enjoy an exercise program.

It's like this. If I told you to pray at 5:00 a.m. every day and you simply couldn't drag yourself out of bed, would this be a reason to not pray at all, or feel less loved by God than someone who is able to do this? I don't think so.

So the takeaway is that you should exercise when you can. And exercise how you like. Try different things from time to time, but if something doesn't work for you, then move on to something else.

I'm going to show you several workout programs. If you've never exercised before, or if it's been a long time since you've exercised regularly, I recommend starting with Program One. If you're more advanced, start with the program that most interests you. I suggest changing routines every four to six weeks, so feel free to switch around and even try new programs from different sources. Again, as long as you stick with the basics, you're going to get results!

A Few Guidelines For Beginners

The most important thing you can do is consult your physician before you start exercising. And if you ever feel faint, dizzy, or anything other than ordinary fatigue while exercising, stop immediately and see a doctor.

I also suggest that you join forces with someone who can show you the proper way to do each exercise. Proper form is crucial to achieving results and minimizing injury. I've provided photos to show you how to perform the exercises (see pages 37–51), but sometimes that isn't enough. My recommendation would be to schedule a few sessions with a certified personal trainer to learn correct exercise execution.

Program 1: Circuit Training

The following program is perfect for the beginning exerciser. If you have little or no training experience, or if you haven't exercised for several months, start here.

This program works the entire body in one workout, two times a week. For the first few weeks, just perform one set of each exercise in the workout. Then change your routine by doing two sets of each exercise for the next few weeks. Finally, do a few weeks of three sets of each exercise. This will build a solid foundation that will prepare your body for more advanced programs.

Your workout should last no longer than one hour. As you add sets to your workouts you'll rest less between sets, so even when you're doing three sets of each exercise you'll be in and out of the gym quickly.

The recommended rest time between sets will depend on your current fitness level. The goal would be to rest no longer than 60 seconds between sets and work to the point where you are moving from one exercise to another with no rest at all.

I've listed all the exercises you should do in the order you should do them. In the Reps column, you'll see how many repetitions of an exercise you should perform in each set. This repetition range will help you determine the amount of weight to use for each exercise. You should use a weight that allows you to perfectly execute at least the minimum recommended number of repetitions, but no more than the maximum recommended number of repetitions. If you're doing leg extensions, for example, and can do 20 repetitions with 100 pounds in perfect form, you're using too light a weight because the maximum recommended number of repetitions is 15.

In the Tempo column, you'll see three numbers. The first number represents the number of seconds it should take you to lift the weight. The second number represents the number of seconds you should hold the weight at the fully contracted position. And the third number represents the number of seconds it should take you to lower the weight.

Circuit-Training Workout

Exercise	Sets	Reps	Tempo
Leg Extension	1-3	12-15	3-0-3
Hamstring Curl	1-3	2-15	3-0-3
Lat Pull Down (To front, reverse grip)	1-3	8-12	3-0-3
Seated Low Row	1-3	8-12	3-0-3
Shoulder Press (Dumbbell or barbell)	1-3	8-12	3-0-3
Lateral Raise	1-3	8-12	3-0-3
Incline Press (Dumbbell or barbell)	1-3	8-12	3-0-3
Flat Bench Press (Dumbbell or barbell)	1-3	8-12	3-0-3
Overhead Dumbbell Extension	1-3	8-12	3-0-3
Press Down (Reverse grip)	1-3	8-12	3-0-3
Bicep Curl (Barbell)	1-3	8-12	3-0-3
Seated Hammer Curl	1-3	8-12	3-0-3
Seated Calf Raise	1-3	12-20	3-1-3
Standing Calf Raise	3-4	6-10	3-1-3
Basic Crunch*	3-4	10-15	3-1-3

* *My Chisel Your Abs video contains valuable information on abdominal training. It's available at www.clarkbartram.com.*

Follow your circuit-training workout with up to 30 minutes of cardiovascular work. Run on a treadmill, walk outside, hop on a StairMaster, or do any activity that elevates your heartbeat to 70% of your maximum heart rate. If you don't know this number, you can calculate it using the following formula:

(220 — Your Age) x .70 = Target Heart Rate

I highly recommend using a heart rate monitor so you can make sure you're exercising at your target heart rate. When you're doing cardiovascular exercise, it doesn't matter how fast you're moving as much as it matters how hard your heart is working. Be careful not to go too far above your target heart rate, especially if you haven't exercised for a long time.

Again, please consult a physician if you have any questions or concerns.

Program 2: Two-Day Split

The following program is suitable for intermediate or advanced exercisers. You'll train upper body on Monday and Thursday and lower body on Tuesday and Friday. Wednesday, Saturday, and Sunday will be your days off. If you feel like doing something on the weekends, choose a cardiovascular activity like walking or rollerblading.

If you're interested in getting bigger muscles, or muscular hypertrophy, follow the recommended rep scheme. If you're more interested in toning and endurance, perform between 12 and 20 repetitions in each set with a lighter weight.

2-Day Split Monday Workout — Chest & Back

Exercise	Sets	Reps	Tempo
Incline Press (Barbell or dumbbell)	3-4	8-12	3-0-3
Lat Pull Down (Reverse grip)	3-4	8-12	3-0-3
Flat Bench Press (Barbell or dumbbell)	3-4	8-12	3-0-3
Lat Pull Down (To front, with wide grip)	3-4	8-12	3-0-3
Dips	1-2	as many as you can	10-0-10*
Seated Low Row (Elbows out)	3-4	8-12	3-0-3

Dips should be performed at a much slower tempo.

2-Day Split Tuesday Workout — Quadriceps & Calves

Exercise	Sets	Reps	Tempo
Squat	3-4	8-12	5-0-5
Leg Press	3-4	8-12	5-0-5
Walking Lunge	2-3	20-30 yards	N/A
Leg Extension	2-3	8-12	5-0-5
Standing Calf Raise	4-6	5-10	5-0-5

2-Day Split Thursday Workout — Shoulders & Arms

Exercise	Sets	Reps	Tempo
Shoulder Press	3-4	8-12	3-0-3
(Dumbbell or barbell)			
Lateral Raise	3-4	8-12	3-0-3
Bent-Over Dumbbell Raise	3-4	8-12	3-0-3
Overhead Dumbbell Extension	3-4	8-12	4-0-4
Bicep Curl	3-4	8-12	4-0-4
(Barbell)			
Bench Dips	2-3	8-12	5-0-5
(Use weight on lap)			
Seated Hammer Curl	2-3	8-12	3-0-3

2-Day Split Friday Workout — Hamstrings & Calves

Exercise	Sets	Reps	Tempo
Hamstring Curl	3-4	8-12	5-0-5
Seated Hamstring Curl	3-4	8-12	3-0-3
Seated Calf Raise	2-3	15-30	3-0-3

2-Day Split/Every Other Day — Abdominals

Perform these extra abdominal exercises after your regular exercises on Mondays and Thursdays or Tuesdays and Fridays.

Exercise	Sets	Reps	Tempo
Swiss Ball Crunch*	3-4	12-20	3-1-3
Leg Raises	3-4	5-10	3-0-3

* *Swiss balls are available at www.clarkbartram.com.*

Program 3: One Body Part a Day

The following program is suitable for intermediate or advanced exercisers. You'll train one body part each day for five straight days, and then take two days off. On every training day, you'll also throw in a couple sets for either calves or abdominals, and you can decide when to include your aerobic activity.

As always, train with intensity and focus, and pay close attention to proper form for each exercise. You should never let momentum help you lift or lower a weight — always follow the tempo recommendations and maintain complete control over the weights you lift.

If you're interested in getting bigger muscles, or muscular hypertrophy, follow the recommended rep scheme. If you're more interested in toning and endurance, perform between 12 and 20 repetitions in each set with a lighter weight.

One Body Part Per Day Monday Workout — Chest

Exercise	Sets	Reps	Tempo
Flat Bench Press	3-4	8-12	3-0-3
(Dumbbell or barbell)			
Incline Press	3-4	8-12	3-0-3
(Dumbbell or barbell)			
Dumbbell Fly	3-4	8-12	5-0-5
Dips	2-3	as many as you can	10-0-10*

Dips should be performed at a much slower tempo.

One Body Part Per Day Tuesday Workout — Back

Exercise	Sets	Reps	Tempo
Bent Row	2	8-12	2-0-2
Pull-Ups	3	as many as you can	3-0-3
(One set each: reverse, prone, and neutral grips)			
Pull Down	3-4	8-12	4—0-4
(Reverse grip)			
Seated Low Row	3-4	8-12	4-0-4

One Body Part Per Day Wednesday Workout — Legs

Exercise	Sets	Reps	Tempo
Squat	3-4	8-10	5-0-5
Leg Press	3-4	8-10	5-0-5
Hack Squat	2-3	8-10	5-0-5
Walking Lunge	1-2	30 yards	N/A
Hamstring Curl (Prone or seated)	3-4	8-10	3-0-3

One Body Part Per Day Thursday Workout — Shoulders

Exercise	Sets	Reps	Tempo
Shoulder Press	3-4	8-12	3-0-3
Upright Row (Wide grip)	3-4	8-12	2-0-2
Lateral Raise	3-4	8-10	3-0-3
Bent-Over Dumbbell Raise	3-4	8-10	2-0-2

One Body Part Per Day Friday Workout — Arms

Exercise	Sets	Reps	Tempo
Overhead Dumbbell Extension	3-4	8-12	5-0-5
Bicep Curl (Barbell)	3-4	8-12	3-0-3
Dips (Elbows tight to body)	2	as many as you can	10-0-10*
Reverse Curl	2-3	8-12	3-0-3
Press Down (Reverse grip)	3-4	8-12	3-0-3

* Dips should be performed at a much slower tempo.

One Body Part Per Day/Every Other Day — Abdominals
Perform these extra abdominal exercises after your regular exercises on alternating days.

Exercise	Sets	Reps	Tempo
Swiss Ball Crunch*	3-4	12-20	3-1-3
Leg Raises	3-4	5-10	3-0-3

* Swiss balls are available at www.clarkbartram.com.

One Body Part Per Day/Every Other Day — Calves

Perform these extra calf exercises after your regular exercises on alternating days when you're not doing extra abdominal work.

Exercise	Sets	Reps	Tempo
Standing Calf Raise	4-6	5-10	5-0-5
Seated Calf Raise	2-3	15-30	3-0-3

The Exercises

All of the exercises recommended in the three workout programs are shown on the following pages, organized by body part. There are many more exercises that you can try as you progress in your fitness lifestyle, but these basic movements should be the foundation of your exercise regimen.

When performing each exercise, be sure to focus on your breathing. Do not hold your breath while lifting weights! Exhale on the lifting, or concentric phase, and inhale on the lowering, or eccentric phase. Novice lifters often use momentum to help lift a weight, but this is cheating and could cause injury. Don't worry about the amount of weight you can lift. It's a lot better to lift a lighter weight with perfect form than it is to lift more weight with momentum. During each exercise, lift the weight deliberately according to my tempo recommendations, and be sure to focus on the muscle you're exercising to get the most out of each repetition.

Posture is another vital element to getting the most out of your efforts in the gym. When doing a standing exercise, for example, try to maintain correct posture — head over your shoulders, shoulders over your hips, and hips over your ankles. In other words, you should be upright and not leaning forward, back, or to either side. Remember to go at your own pace and exercise hard, but smart. This is a lifestyle now, not a short-term fix to a problem. Develop good habits along the way, and the experience will be both beneficial and fun.

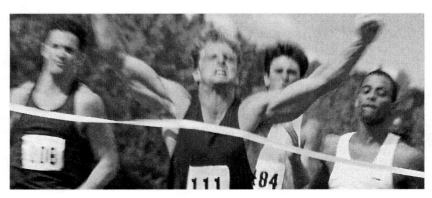

LEGS

Leg Press
Keep your feet about shoulder-width apart. Lower the weight as far as you can without allowing your hips to come off the pad.

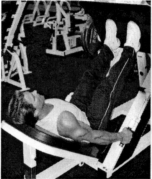 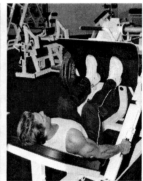

Squat
Keep your feet shoulder-width apart and angled to about 30 degrees. Look straight to the horizon and squat until your thighs are parallel to the floor. Be sure to keep your knees tracking over your toes — do not allow your knees to wander in or out.

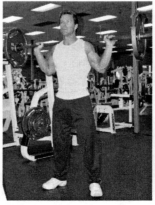 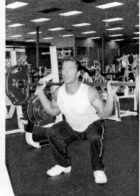

Seated Hamstring Curl

Be sure the machine is adjusted properly and go slowly. With this exercise, a little weight goes a long way!

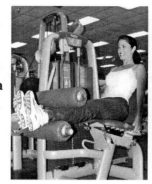
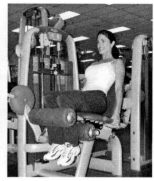

Walking Lunge

Place the weight on your upper shoulders and slowly step forward with one leg, taking a normal stride. Lower yourself slowly until you feel a stretch in your glutes, or butt muscles. Be sure your leading knee stays behind and over your toes, not allowing it to wander in or out. Return to a standing position. For variety, you can do your repetitions one leg at a time while standing in place, with alternate legs from a stationary position, or by walking across the room.

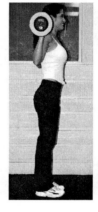
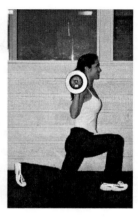

Hamstring Curl

Slowly curl the weight up with your legs. With this exercise, a little weight goes a long way!

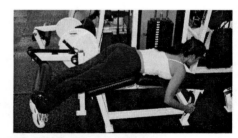
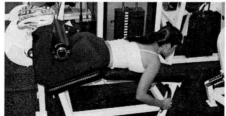

Hack Squat

Adjust your feet for comfort — most people use a shoulder-width stance. Lower yourself slowly to a comfortable position, making sure that your knees stay over your toes.

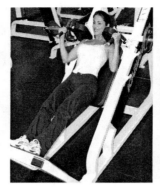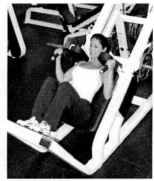

Leg Extension

Be sure that the seat is adjusted so your knees are in line with the axis of the machine. Extend your legs and squeeze your thigh muscles at the top of the movement.

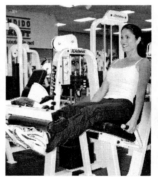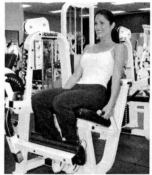

BACK

Pull-Ups

Do as many repetitions as you can with each grip. Don't be discouraged if you can't do many at first, you'll develop the strength over time. If you can't do even one complete pull up, do the eccentric portion only by using a stool to get to the top of the bar and then slowly lowering yourself down.

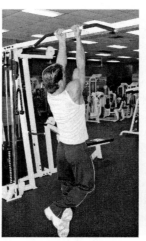 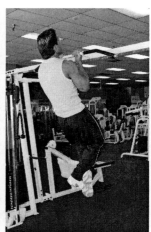

Lat Pull Down

It's much safer to pull to the front of your body. Pull to your upper chest without leaning back.

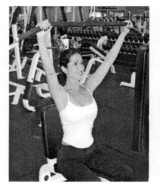 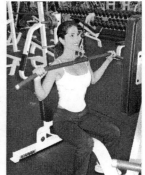

Lat Pull Down

(Reverse Grip)
Using a reverse grip
will help isolate your
lat muscles. Be sure to
get a full range of
motion and don't lean
back.

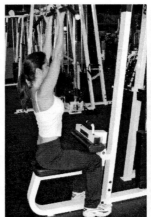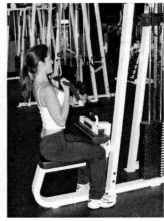

Seated Low Row

Keep a slight bend in
your knees and pull to
your lower chest/upper
abs. Keep your elbows
in tight and don't lean
back or too far forward.

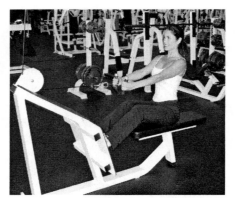

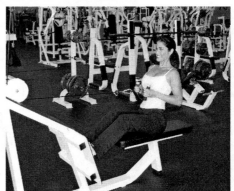

BICEPS

Bicep Curl with Barbell

Stand with good posture and keep your feet about shoulder-width apart. Curl the weight up and contract your biceps. Lower slowly.

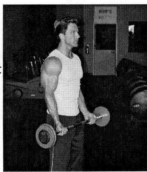 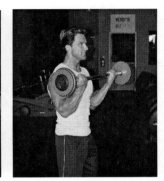

Bicep Curl with Dumbbell

Using dumbbells allows you to curl one arm at a time. This is good because you can see if one arm is stronger than the other. If so, do one additional set on the weaker side.

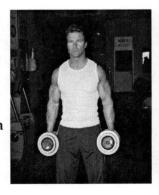 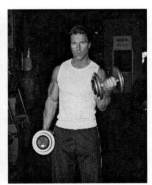

Reverse Curl

Grasp the bar with your arms and feet about shoulder-width apart. Curl up slowly and return. This will work the muscles of your forearm in addition to your biceps.

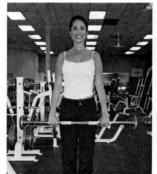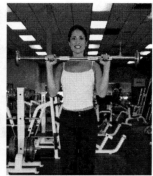

Seated Hammer Curl

Grasp two dumbbells and rotate your hands so that your thumbs are facing the ceiling. Curl up slowly and return.

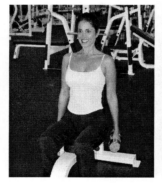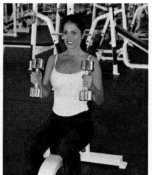

CHEST

Dumbbell Fly

Start by choosing a fairly light set of dumbbells. Carefully lie back on a flat bench and slowly lower the weights to your sides, with elbows slightly bent. Return as if you were hugging a tree.

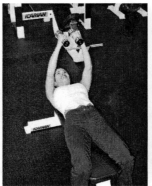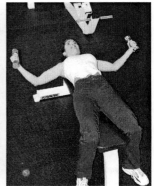

Flat Bench Press

Grasp the bar at a comfortable width and lower to your chest, or at least to the point where your upper arms are parallel to the floor.

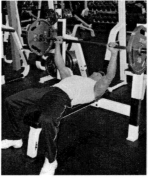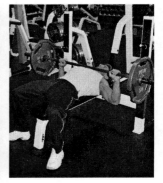

Incline Press (Barbell)

Lower the bar to your upper chest and return.

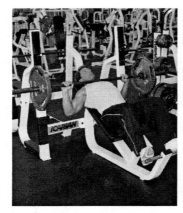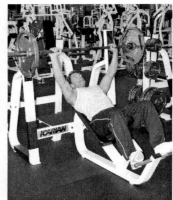

Incline Press (Dumbbell)

Lower the dumbbells to your upper chest/clavicle and return. If you notice that one side is weaker than the other, do one extra set with the weaker side.

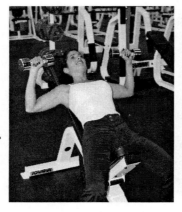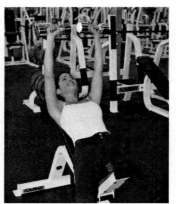

SHOULDERS

Shoulder Press

Press the weight straight up without banging the weights together at the top. Lower slowly.

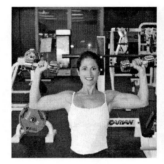 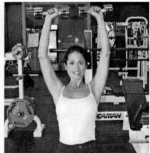

Lateral Raise

Stand with feet shoulder-width apart and raise the weight up with slightly bent elbows until your arms are parallel with the floor.

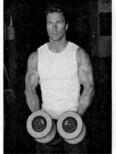 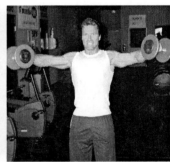

Bent-Over Dumbbell Raise

Bend over with the weights in your hands, knees slightly bent, and feet shoulder-width apart. Concentrate on lifting the weights from the elbows and squeezing your scapula together.

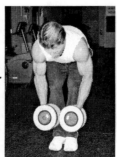 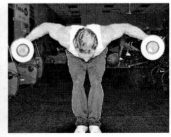

49

TRICEPS

Overhead Dumbbell Extension

This is my favorite triceps exercise. Use a fairly heavy dumbbell and keep your elbows stationary and tight to your ears. Lower as far as you can comfortably go. Return and contract the triceps at the top of the movement.

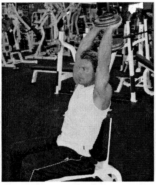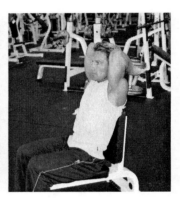

Press Downs (Reverse Grip)

Use a cable machine and select the appropriate weight. With your palms facing up, straighten your arm and squeeze the triceps muscles. Return slowly and be sure to maintain perfect posture.

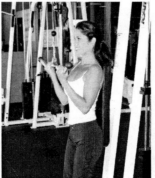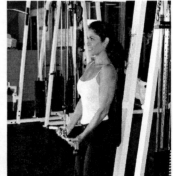

Bench Dips

Using two benches, place your hands on one and your feet on the other. If possible, use a weight on your lap. Lower slowly but not too far — you don't want to over-stretch your deltoid muscles.

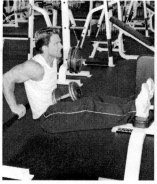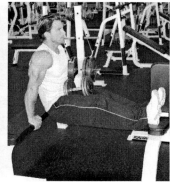

Dips (Elbows In)

This dip exercise can be used for your chest, as well as your triceps. Keeping your elbows tight to the body will emphasize the triceps. Rotating your elbows out will cause your chest to work harder. Just remember to only go as low as your body is comfortable.

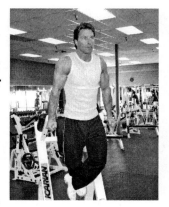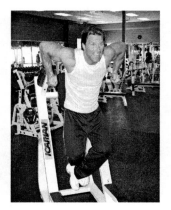

CALVES

Seated Calf Raise

When your knees are bent during a calf exercise, you focus mainly on your soleus muscle. The soleus is made of mainly slow-twitch fibers that respond best to more reps with lighter resistance.

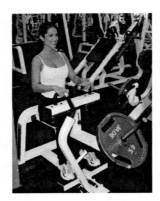 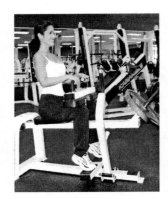

Standing Calf Raise

The standing calf raise exercises the gastroc muscles that are made of mostly fast-twitch fibers. These muscles respond best to fewer reps with more weight.

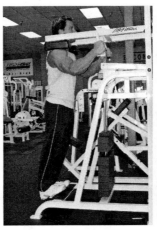 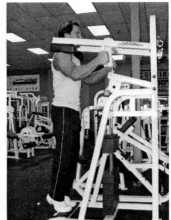

ABDOMINALS

Basic Crunch

Imagine that a helium balloon on your chest is pulling your upper body straight up. Bend only at the waist and remember that this is not a big movement. Exhale on the effort to ensure maximum contraction.

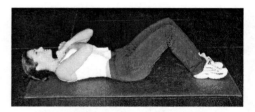
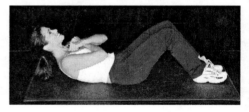

Leg Raises

Start by lying flat on your back with your hands at your sides. Now press your lower back into the floor, lift your legs up about six inches, and lower slowly.

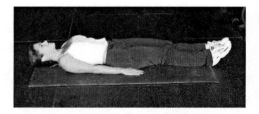
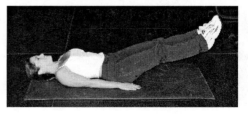

Swiss Ball Crunch

This is my all-time favorite abdominal exercise. Sit on the ball just below the top, towards the front of the ball. Lay back and allow your spine to wrap around the ball. Return to the start position and exhale. Be careful not to fall off the ball!

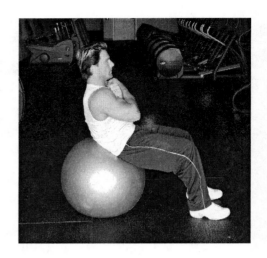

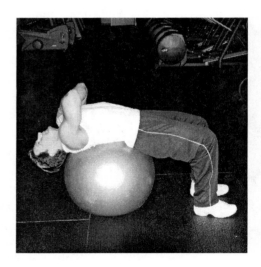

Chapter Six

God's Nutrition Plan for a Lean, Healthy Body

*"I try to avoid looking forward or backward,
and try to keep looking upward!"*

-- Charlotte Bronte

God, in his infinite wisdom, provides all the nutrition we need to maintain a healthy existence. As sources of food, animals and plants give us the three macronutrients we need — protein to build and maintain muscle, carbohydrates for fuel, and fat for healthy skin, hair, and nerves.

In the natural world, God has also given us the micronutrients — vitamins and minerals — that we need in small amounts to release the energy from the whole natural foods we eat. And, of course, He's given us water, which accounts for 70% of the total weight of our bodies and is therefore obviously vital to our health. *(See sidebar on page 92.)*

If we followed God's nutrition plan and only ate a variety of natural foods and only drank water, we wouldn't have many of the health problems that are so common today. We wouldn't have such a prevalence of heart disease, hypertension, diabetes, or obesity. I also believe that we'd appreciate our food more and feel more spiritually connected to the wondrous cycle of Creation.

Where have we missed the mark?

A trip to the supermarket shows how far away we've come from God's nutrition plan. Every time we go to the store, we're tempted by the bright packages and seductive tastes of processed foods — sugary sodas, salty snacks, bleached flour, and fake fats that have no nutritional value. These foods may offer convenience and short-term satisfaction, but they can ultimately result in long-term problems.

Now, I realize that the human ingenuity that came up with all these processed foods is also one of God's blessings, but in these cases I think it's been misused. The good news is that it is possible to find manmade foods that offer convenience, good taste, and good nutrition. Vitamin and mineral supplements are great examples of how people have used God's gifts for the benefit of human health.

I recommend that you take a good multivitamin and mineral supplement every morning. You might even make it part of a spiritual ritual, where you praise God for another glorious day of health and vitality. As you take your supplement each morning, you can offer a prayer of thanks for your life and ask God for continued health.

Food, Glorious Food

But what are you supposed to do the rest of the day? I understand that you have a busy schedule, social obligations, and other commitments that get in the way of good eating. And it's not like we have time to hunt our own meat and pick our own berries.

But there are ways to avoid running into a fast food restaurant or skipping meals altogether, both of which do a disservice to the body.

I believe that when you have an attitude of praise for God's creation, you'll naturally want to eat better. Not only for yourself, but for your family, your co-workers, your church, and all the other people who are sharing God's bounty with you as you live your life.

And it's okay to take small steps toward better eating. Maybe you'll have a plain grilled chicken sandwich instead of a double cheeseburger. Maybe you'll bring some raw vegetables and nuts to snack on at the office if you can't leave your desk. Maybe you'll go to the supermarket and only pick one or two items out of the snack aisle.

As human beings, none of us are perfect, and it's not fair to tell yourself you have to start eating perfectly right away. You'll just feel guilty if you don't live up to your lofty standards. Just start taking a God perspective when it comes to eating and shopping for food and see what happens.

How Much Can I Eat?

More people ask me how much they can eat than any other question when it comes to nutrition. And let me tell you, that's not an easy one to answer! The Bible says that you are a unique creation made by God. There's no one else in the entire world with your laugh, your facial features, your fingerprints (thank God for that one), your mannerisms, or your personality.

When I look at my kids and see the difference in their personalities, I wonder how they came from the same set of parents. One is gentle and quiet, while the other is wild and full of energy. When I compare myself to my brothers, I'm amazed at how different we are. My "little" brother is 5'11," weighs 265 pounds, and is as tough as can be, while I'm 5'8," weigh 190 pounds, and avoid conflict at all costs.

Now, you may be wondering to yourself,
"What does all this have to do with nutrition?"

The answer is — EVERYTHING! Since you are a unique creation made by God, the amount of food you can eat is going to be different from everyone else's. I believe this is why America's obsession with losing weight has been so frustrating over the years. People believe the incredible claims of fad diets that promise a lean, muscular physique in as little as 48 hours! While some folks may benefit from the different diets in the marketplace today, the majority of people don't get the fantastic results described in the enticing advertisements. The diet marketers get rich, and millions of people feel like failures and may end up believing that they'll never be able to lose weight.

Americans spend nearly 50 billion dollars each year in an attempt to lose weight, and each year the obese population in our country increases. It doesn't take a rocket scientist to see that the fad diet approach to effective weight loss is seriously wrong!

Now, this still doesn't tell you how much you can eat in order to get your best body. I have to be honest when I say that this book has been pretty much of a breeze to write except for this chapter. This is actually the fourth rewrite of what could very well be the "make-it-or-break-it" section of my book. I showed the first drafts of this chapter to friends and family members, and each time some of them came back to me and said, "I tried that and it didn't work for me," or "I did that and then gained the weight right back."

So here's what I decided. I'm going to tell you what's worked for me, and I'm also going to give you some general guidelines that you can start applying as you learn what works for you.

These general guidelines start with the idea that whole foods are a whole lot better than processed foods for transforming your body. Like I said earlier, God has given us all we need in the natural world to sustain ourselves and maintain good health, so if you can begin there it'll be easier to make further modifications that will dramatically change your body.

Optimal Nutrition for Your Body

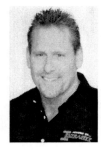

In 1997 I met William Smith, the CEO/President of INTRAFITT Corporation. He's been helping people meet their individual nutritional needs for more than a dozen years. Since we met, his Three Elements of Optimal Nutrition have been the cornerstone of my nutrition program, and I'm confident that they can help you determine what dietary changes will work for you. I enlisted his help in writing this chapter because I wanted to give you the best information possible. Most of what you'll read about nutrition on the following pages comes directly from his years of experience creating individualized nutrition programs that get results for thousands of people across the country and around the world.

According to William, anyone — regardless of his or her existing condition — can reprogram his or her body to be fit, lean, healthy, and strong for the rest of his or her life with a basic and general understanding of what, when, and how to eat. Why spend another day feeling anything but optimal?!

I'd like to point out that "Optimal" Nutrition means much more than simply eating whole natural foods. Optimal Nutrition means eating the correct number of calories, the correct ratio of energy nutrients (protein, carbohydrates, and fats), and the correct number of meals throughout the day for your body's individual needs.

Optimal Nutrition Element One — Proper Calorie Intake

Are we finally going to answer the question of how much you can eat? Like I said before, the answer is going to be different for everyone reading this book, but I can give you a few guidelines.

First of all, you need to know that if you eat too many calories at any one sitting and/or throughout the day, your body is likely to store the excess energy in the form of body fat. That's not a hard concept to grasp.

But did you realize that the opposite is also true?! If you don't eat enough calories at any given meal and/or throughout the day (such as when you follow a calorie-restricted diet or simply miss a meal because you're too busy), you actually program your body to store fat much more efficiently, thereby making it harder to lose body fat. So the key is finding the exact number of calories you can eat so your body doesn't store fat.

You may be aware that many diets tell you how many calories you're supposed to eat in a day. But if you think about it, we don't eat day-to-day —

we eat meal-to-meal. Therefore, your question should really be "How many calories should I be eating at each meal, and how many meals should I be eating each day?

There exists a specific calorie intake — per meal — that best suits your body's individual metabolic variables. Metabolic variables include your age, height, gender, total body weight, body composition, current activity level, current type of activity, current eating habits, genetics, and desired health & fitness goals. As you can see, there are a number of factors that determine the amount of food you should be eating for Optimal Nutrition. That's what makes figuring out how much you can eat so complicated!

For a specific recommendation, you can visit www.clarkbartram.com, click the "Nutrition" link, and order an individualized nutrition program from INTRAFITT. Or you can experiment on your own. Write down everything you eat and when you eat it for two or three days. You'll see if you're missing meals or eating too much or too little at one sitting. You'll see if you're eating too many processed foods. You'll then want to modify your diet so that you're eating balanced meals consisting of naturally-occurring protein, carbohydrates, and fats every three or four hours, but we'll get into that a little bit later.

First, I want to talk about the nutrients that are important for a healthy diet.

Powerful Protein

Protein is the most abundant element in the body next to water and plays a vital role in the development and maintenance of your body's enzymes, hormones, hemoglobin, skin, hair, nails, muscles, and even antibodies. Protein can also be used as an energy source by the body.

Protein is available in two forms, complete and incomplete. Complete proteins are derived from animal sources such as fish, poultry, beef, eggs, milk, and cheese. Incomplete proteins are derived from plants such as nuts, seeds, and grains.

Proteins are considered complete when they contain all of the essential amino acids that your body needs. Complete proteins also have a more profound affect on the hormones that influence the breakdown of fats within the body. Incomplete proteins do not have all the essential amino acids, and therefore they can't be used as efficiently as complete proteins.

I recommend eating up to one gram of protein per pound of lean body weight. To find out what your lean body weight is, visit www.clarkbartram.com and click on the online body fat calculator. There are about 30 grams of protein in a boneless, skinless chicken breast and about 14 grams of protein in a serving of cottage cheese. Protein bars or powder supplements vary widely, so read the labels.

Fuel Up With Carbohydrates

Carbohydrates are the body's chief source of fuel, and are the exclusive fuel source for the brain and nervous system. Although carbs are getting a bad wrap these days, they play an essential role in the fat-burning process and should be included at every meal.

The problem with carbohydrates is that when you eat too many of them at once, they can release excessive levels of insulin in the bloodstream. High insulin levels have been linked to a number of chronic and degenerative diseases such as obesity, diabetes, and coronary heart disease. Carbohydrates can be divided into two groups — simple and complex. Simple carbohydrates release a lot of insulin quickly, and complex carbohydrates release less insulin at a slower rate. Most people are aware that simple carbohydrates include fruits, juices, candy, pastries, sodas, and sugar, but many people don't know that pasta, potatoes, cereals, carrots, and rice are simple carbohydrates, too. Better sources of carbohydrates include oats, sweet potatoes, green vegetables, and apples.

The Skinny On Fat

Dietary fats are equally important in the metabolic windmill. Unfortunately, people associate dietary fats with the fat they want to lose around their hips, thighs, and buttocks. In most cases, excessive body fat is not a result of eating too much dietary fat, but rather from eating too many refined sugars and processed foods and not exercising enough. In fact, eating naturally-derived fats such as nuts, olives, and avocados is a lot less likely to make you fat than eating refined and processed sugars because of the insulin response associated with these foods.

Naturally-derived dietary fats are helpful in the following ways:

- Dietary fats help to prolong the emptying time of the stomach after a meal, therefore increasing satiety (the feeling of fullness)
- Dietary fats help regulate the release of insulin, thereby suppressing the rate at which triglycerides are formed within the fat cells of the body
- Dietary fats provide essential fatty acids that are critical for normal growth, a healthy circulatory and nervous system, and for keeping the skin and other tissues of the body fit and youthful.

Consider adding a little flaxseed oil to your salads or taking an Omega-3 fatty acid supplement.

Vitamins and Minerals

Vitamin and minerals are micronutrients that the body uses to release the energy from food. They're important components of your diet, but The Anarem Report has shown that not one person out of more than 21,000 people surveyed received the U.S. RDA (Recommended Daily Allowance) of magnesium, calcium, iron, and vitamins B1, B2, B6, B12, and C. Take a good multivitamin and mineral supplement each day.

Water

Drink plenty of water instead of coffee, soda, or juice. Active individuals should drink a minimum of 1.5 gallons of water each day. See page 92 for ten good reasons why you should drink a lot of water.

Sports Drinks

Sports drinks are useful when consumed after or during vigorous and prolonged exercise in high heat. But most experts agree that water works better with moderate exercise.

Supplements

Even though I've been a paid spokesperson for supplement companies in the past and am now promoting my own supplement line, I've always chosen the "high road" in answering questions about supplements. Bottom line — there's no magic pill or secret sauce in the supplement world. There's no replacement for hard work and great eating habits, but there are some very useful and valid supplements on the market today. Not everyone is out to rip off your hard-earned dollars.

As I mentioned earlier, I believe that everyone needs to be on a high-quality multi-vitamin and mineral supplement to compensate for things like missed meals or depleted soils. This type of supplementation provides a solid foundation, kind of like building your house on rock and not sand.

Secondly, I highly suggest some kind of joint support supplementation like chondroitin sulfate and glucosamine. Regardless of how regularly we work out, at some point we'll begin to feel the effects of aging on the joints of our body. I think that it's wise to keep them healthy with a little preventive maintenance.

Third, if you absolutely have no way to access "real food," a great-tasting, well-balanced meal replacement powder (MRP) is a better choice than a skipped meal. Just make sure that the protein source in your MRP is derived from high-grade whey.

There are many other supplements on the market for specific conditions, designed to do things like improve your vision, help you sleep better, or ease you through menopause. I believe that many of these all-natural products can be effective, and I suggest that you do your own research to become a more educated consumer. A great place to start is www.clarkbartram.com and check out my new supplement line designed specifically to meet the needs of the "everyday" person such as yourself. I plan to expand the line as demand grows for new and innovative, scientifically based products.

Optimal Nutrition Element Two — Proper Nutrient Ratios

Now that we have a basic idea of what and how much you should be eating, we can move on to INTRAFITT's second element of Optimal Nutrition.

The nutrient composition of each meal you eat, along with the specific way you exercise, orchestrates hormonal responses that ultimately determine whether you burn excess body fat for energy, or store it on your hips, thighs, buttocks, stomach, or other undesirable locations. Without a clear understanding of how to eat in order to control these hormonal responses, long-term fat loss will forever remain an elusive goal.

Let's say that your individual calorie recommendation is 520 cal/meal.

There are lots of ways to eat 520 calories, and it's quite possible that one combination of nutrients may lead to a favorable change in body composition while another combination could have an adverse effect.

Meal #1 — Muscle Gain		Meal #2 — Fat Gain	
Food	*Calories*	*Food*	*Calories*
6 oz. chicken breast (protein)	186	8 oz. chicken breast (protein)	248
7 oz. yams (carbohydrate)	210	2 oz. yams (carbohydrate)	60
3 oz. broccoli (carbohydrate)	24	1.5 oz. broccoli (carbohydrate)	12
1 tbs. peanut butter (fat)	100	2 tbs. peanut butter (fat)	200
Total Calories	520	Total Calories	520

As you can see, even a slight change in nutrient ratios can have an impact on the hormonal responses that can give you your best body!

When putting meals together, the easiest thing to do is to choose one portion of protein, one portion of carbohydrate, and one portion of fat. I tell people never to eliminate any type of food — like carbohydrates or fats — in an effort to lose weight quickly. By choosing one portion of each of the energy nutrients, you'll be able to create balanced meals that are nutritious and delicious, and that are likely to create positive hormonal responses that result in fat loss and muscle gain.

Use the following guidelines to determine the right portion sizes:

Nutrient	Portion Size Equals
Carbohydrate	Size of Clenched Fist
Protein	Size of the Palm of Your Hand
Fat	Size of the Top Knuckle to the Tip of Your Thumb

Then choose a portion from each category in the chart below to create your balanced meals throughout the day:

Protein	Carbohydrate	Fat
Chicken	Red Potatoes	Avocado
Fish	Sweet potatoes	Almonds
Turkey	Yams	Olive Oil
Eggs	Summer Squash	Fish Oils
Tofu	Oatmeal	Essential Fatty Acids
Lean Beef	Brown Rice	Egg Yolks (if limited)
Buffalo	7-Grain Bread	Safflower Mayonnaise
Ostrich	Pasta	Butter (real)
Lean Pork	Cantaloupe	
Egg Substitute	Broccoli	
Canned Chicken Breast	Green Beans	
Canned Tuna	Spinach/Greens	
Lean Ham	Pinto Beans	
Low Fat Cottage Cheese	Whole Wheat Tortillas	
Protein Powder		
Shrimp		

This portion-control system has worked well for me, and it should be a great way for you to start following God's nutrition plan. You'll inevitably feel better, have more energy, and begin to see rapid and favorable changes in your body.

For incredibly tasty meal ideas, see My Favorite Recipes starting on page 64.

Optimal Nutrition Element Three — Meal Intervals

After you eat a balanced meal made up of protein, carbohydrates, and fats, your body can sustain blood sugar levels above baseline normal for approximately three or four hours.

If your blood sugar drops below normal, you may experience sugar cravings, headaches, lethargy (tiredness), shakiness, agitation, and even depression or anxiety. Low blood sugar, or hypoglycemia, can result from a number of different situations, the most common being waiting too long to eat between meals, eating food that is disproportionately high in sugar, eating highly refined and processed foods, or the repeated subjection to a restricted-calorie diet. Needless to say, hypoglycemia is one of the most common nutrition-related problems in America. Hypoglycemia is one of the major problems with most approaches to dieting in this country, because anytime the body is purposely starved in an effort to lose weight rapidly it initiates thousands of biochemical reactions that will at some point become so strong, no amount of willpower in the world can overcome them. As a result, people on diets often binge on sugary foods to satisfy their intense cravings.

This entire process is often followed by self-abuse, which exacerbates an already existing distortion of self-image. The tendency is to want to immediately starve the body once again, creating a vicious circle of self-destruction.

The way around this is to eat a balanced meal containing protein, carbohydrates, and fat every three or four hours throughout the day. If you wake up at 6:00 a.m. and eat your first meal within one hour, for example, you would then eat your next meal between 10:00 a.m. and 11:00 a.m. in order to maintain normal blood sugar levels. If you continued with this schedule throughout the rest of the day, you'd end up eating about five meals before you go to bed. If you stay up late one night, you could feasibly need to eat a total of six meals in one day. If you sleep in one day, you may only need to eat three or four meals. This is okay, because the recommended meal interval for Optimal Nutrition is three or four hours from within one hour of waking to within one hour of going to sleep. While you sleep, your blood sugar levels drop and you're in a hypoglycemic state when you wake up in the morning. That's why you should never exercise in the morning on an empty stomach. You'll end up losing weight, but it will be in the form of water and muscle protein! You're also likely to feel tired and sluggish, crave sugar, and risk the onset of headaches, depression, and agitation throughout the day.

Personally, I eat six properly structured meals each day. You may find, however, that eating four meals per day (one meal every four hours or so) works best for you! If you find yourself out and about without access to a properly balanced meal, the following snack items are great blood sugar boosters that can tide you over until you can eat a good meal:

- Piece of Fruit
- Protein Bar (I really don't like these but they're better than nothing)
- Raw Veggies
- Low-Fat Cottage Cheese with Fruit
- Celery and Almond Butter
- Air-Popped Popcorn

- Plain Yogurt
- Almonds or Cashews (be careful here —
  no more than a small handful)
- Cheese Stick and Apple

There are many other acceptable snacks, but this list should do the trick.

Nobody's Perfect

As I mentioned before, striving for perfect eating habits is admirable, but demanding it from yourself only leads to guilt and frustration. Life is here to be enjoyed, so if you like a glass of wine now and then or have a special place in your heart for chocolate ice cream, it's okay to indulge on occasion.

Once or twice a week, treat yourself to something special like a slice of pizza or a piece of cake. It will only help you appreciate the fact that you're following God's nutrition plan the rest of the time.

To stay on course, think of three reasons why you want to improve the way you eat. Then write them down and make copies. Post the copies on your bathroom mirror, on your refrigerator, near the television set, and next to your bed as a constant reminder of the "Commitment to Excellence" that you've made to yourself and to God. Then each day, reaffirm this commitment in your mind and in your heart and remember that you and only you have the ability to live each day of your life fulfilled with energy, strength, vitality, understanding, forgiveness, and, above all, gratefulness.

Remember, "Optimal Nutrition" is about giving your body, mind, and soul the exact amount of whole natural food you need to give back to this earth what this earth has given to you. Don't take this commitment lightly, as the days of your life in this world are limited and God is relying on you. Remember, Spiritual Fitness begins from within, which is what the INTRAFITT philosophy is all about.

Food — A Christian Perspective

Many Christians associate food with guilt and weakness. After all, Eve gave in to the temptation of food in the Garden of Eden. But God is a lot smarter than the devil, and it is possible to view food as the nourishment and sustenance that it was meant to be. Remember, the same thing the devil used to tempt Eve is what God used at the Last Supper to bring people into communion with Him.

My Favorite Recipes

Below you'll find a few of my favorite things to eat. Most are pretty easy to prepare and take with you while you're out running around all day. That's half the battle — you must be prepared when you're out of the house for the day. Discover some fast and easy recipes of your own and always remember to be prepared or you'll end up in a drive-thru somewhere!

Barbeque Egg Burrito

1 medium flour or whole-wheat tortilla
6 eggs, only 2 yolks
Smokin' Joe Jones Barbeque sauce
Cook eggs, warm tortilla, add sauce and eggs on tortilla and eat.
I was getting tired of my regular burrito and decided to try this one. It may sound weird, but it's great!

Vanilla Oatmeal

1 serving of whole oats (one handful, dry)
1 teaspoon vanilla
Dash of cinnamon
1 scoop vanilla protein powder
Cook oatmeal, add vanilla, cinnamon, and protein powder (use extra water to absorb the protein powder), and eat. You'll need to experiment with amounts a bit.

Yam & Peanut Butter

1 medium yam
1 tablespoon natural peanut or almond butter
Pierce the yam several times with a fork. Microwave for 6-8 minutes.
Add peanut butter after the yam is cooked. This is a great treat!

Chicken Sandwich
6-8 oz. canned (Tyson-brand) chicken breast
1 tablespoon safflower mayonnaise
2 pieces 7-grain bread
Lowry's Season Salt
Avocado
Combine safflower mayonnaise with chicken, toast bread, spread chicken mixture on bread, add avocado, and sprinkle with seasoning.

Spicy Chicken Burrito
One store-bought rotisserie chicken
Hot sauce
1 medium flour or whole-wheat tortilla
Brown all the meat from the chicken in a pan lined with Pam® cooking spray; add hot sauce while cooking. (I know the chicken is already cooked!) Heat tortilla, fill with ingredients, wrap, and eat. This can be made with barbeque or teriyaki sauce, too.

Turkey Patties
93% fat-free ground turkey breast
Italian-flavored bread crumbs
Combine ingredients, fry in a pan lined with Pam® cooking spray, and eat with a side of raw or cooked green beans.

Anita's Spinach Salad
1 cup pine nuts
1 pound spinach, washed and crisped
2 cups cauliflower flowerets
1 large, ripe avocado
Lemon juice
6 tablespoons olive oil
2 tablespoons white wine vinegar
1 large garlic clove, minced or pressed
1/4 tablespoon each of salt, dry mustard, and dry basil
1 teaspoon pepper
Dash of nutmeg
Toast nuts over medium heat in a small frying pan, shaking the pan

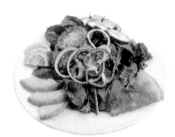

often until the nuts are golden brown. Set aside. Remove and throw away spinach stems. Tear large leaves into bite-sized pieces. Slice cauliflower into bite-sized pieces, as well.

Pit, peel, and slice the avocado; coat slices in lemon juice. Combine with spinach and cauliflower in a large bowl. In a separate, smaller bowl, combine the oil, vinegar, garlic, salt, mustard, basil, pepper, and nutmeg. Mix until well blended.

Pour dressing over salad, add nuts, and mix lightly.

TIP: Add some rotisserie-cooked chicken to make this salad a meal.

Healthy Turkey Pot Pie
(from Chef Miki Knowles)
1 15-oz. package of pie crusts, refrigerated
1/3 cup veggie butter
1/3 cup onion, chopped
1/3 cup all-purpose flour
1/2 teaspoon salt
1/4 teaspoon pepper
1-1/2 cups chicken broth
2/3 cup veggie milk
1-1/2 pounds turkey, diced
10 oz. frozen mixed vegetables

Pre-heat your oven to 425 degrees. Prepare piecrusts as directed on package for a two-crust pie using a 9-inch pie pan. In a medium saucepan, melt veggie butter, add onion, and cook two minutes until tender. Stir in flour, salt, and pepper. Gradually stir in broth and veggie milk. Cook the mixture, stirring constantly until bubbly and thickened. Add turkey and mixed vegetables and remove from heat. Spoon the turkey mixture into a crust-lined pan. Top with second crust and seal edges together — cut slits in several places. Bake the pie at 425 degrees for 35 minutes or until crust is golden brown. Let stand for 5 minutes prior to serving. Serves eight.

Thai Turkey Roll-Ups
(from Chef Miki Knowles)
1 tablespoon lime juice
1 tablespoon light mayonnaise
1 teaspoon reduced-fat peanut butter
1/4 teaspoon ground red pepper
1 teaspoon ground ginger

1 garlic clove, crushed
2 10-inch flour tortillas
1/4 cup chopped fresh basil
2 large Napa (Chinese) cabbage leaves
3 oz. thinly sliced deli-roasted turkey breast
1/2 cup red bell pepper strips
Combine the first six ingredients in a bowl, stirring well with a whisk. Spread each tortilla with one tablespoon of the mayonnaise mixture. Top each tortilla with two tablespoons of basil, one cabbage leaf, half of the sliced turkey breast, and half of the bell peppers. Roll up, wrap in plastic wrap, and chill in refrigerator. Serves four.

Chocolate Chip Pound Cake

3/4 cup veggie butter
1 cup sugar
1 teaspoon orange rind, grated
1 teaspoon vanilla
4 eggs
2 cups flour
1 teaspoon baking powder
1/2 teaspoon salt
1/2 cup veggie milk
1/2 cup semisweet chocolate chips
Preheat oven to 325 degrees. With an electric mixer, cream the veggie butter and sugar until light and fluffy. Mix in the orange rind and vanilla. Add eggs, one at a time, beating well after each addition. Mix flour, baking powder, and salt in a separate bowl and slowly add the flour mixture to the veggie butter mixture. Beat until well-blended, then fold in the chocolate chips. Spread into a greased and floured 9" x 5" loaf pan. Bake about 60 – 75 minutes, or until a wooden pick inserted in the center comes out clean. Let stand in the pan for 10 minutes, then turn out onto a rack to complete cooling. Serves eight.

Stuffed Peppers

Green, yellow, and red peppers
93% fat free turkey breast
Rice
Tomato sauce

Cut peppers in half, boil until soft, and brown turkey meat in separate pan. Cook rice completely. Combine meat and rice and stuff into pepper halves. Line in a cooking dish, cover with tomato sauce, and bake for about 40-50 minutes. These are great little compact meals complete with all the necessary macronutrients.

I hope you enjoy these recipes as much as I do! If you're looking for more great recipes, log on to my television show's Web site at **www.amerfit.com** and click on Peak Nutrition.

Chapter Seven

Resisting Temptation

"If you can find a path with no obstacles, it probably doesn't lead anywhere."

-- Frank A. Clark

Now that you know everything you need to get a fit and healthy body that will enrich your spirit, all you have to do is put it into practice by eating right, going to the gym regularly, and keeping a positive attitude. Easier said than done, right? Just like keeping your faith alive, getting and staying in shape requires discipline.

There are many things along the path to physical fitness that will try to lead you astray. Here are some tips to help you resist temptation and remain true to your pursuit of physical and spiritual well-being. Some of the suggestions might seem basic and maybe you've even heard them before, but believe me, they can be valuable tools if you find that "living the lifestyle" is becoming a struggle.

1. Like yourself now.

People with low self-esteem are often the first to give into temptation. They expect immediate results, and if things don't change right away they tend to despair and feel like their goals are unattainable, so they simply give up. Everyone's journey on this earth is different, and the path to spiritual and physical balance is often a long one. And believe it or not, it's really not so much about results as it is about making the effort and having the confidence to persevere. I've seen people get into great shape and still remain unhappy with themselves — happiness is not a superficial issue. You can strengthen your resolve and learn to like yourself by realizing that you are a unique creation of a God who loves you. Fortify your fitness regimen with the confidence that comes from a strong faith, and use the affirmations we talked about on page XX to keep yourself on track.

2. Learn to recognize

all the lame excuses you're going to use to avoid exercising. "It's raining out." "I'm tired." "I'm busy." "The car won't start." "The gym's too crowded at five o'clock." "I have to work late." These are not legitimate excuses to skip a workout. If you can't get to the gym, you can exercise at home, go for a walk or a run, jump rope, do some pushups, etc. If the President of the United States can find time to exercise, so can you! Sometimes you'll have a good reason to skip a workout, but as soon as you start making excuses ask yourself if they're really legitimate.

3. Choose an accountability partner.

I believe that "you're only committed to what you confess," in faith as well as in fitness. That's why it's good to have someone with an understanding ear to talk to about your successes and failures as you pursue health and fitness. Find someone you can trust and tell them what you want to accomplish, and what your concerns and fears are. For example, you might tell this person that you want to lose 20 pounds in three months, but you have a weakness for chocolate chip cookies. This person can be a professional trainer or nutritionist, a life coach, a like-minded member of your congregation, a friend, or even a family member. Whoever you choose (and you may have more than one person), they should be ready at all times to share your achievements and help you when you have a problem or an emergency. They should be someone you could call while you're walking down the cookie aisle in the grocery store!

4. Don't go grocery shopping when you're hungry!

You're much more likely to give in to your particular food cravings and be tempted by the attractive packaging of processed foods.

5. Don't do fad diets!

They might work for the short term, but most people gain the weight back later. I'd rather see you learn how to portion your food correctly instead of depriving your body of particular nutrients. See pages XX–XX for details.

6. Don't eat in front of the television.

People who eat in front of the tube generally overeat. This occurs partly because concentrating on a program makes you unaware of all the food your shoveling into your mouth, and partly because stimulating food advertising makes you think you're hungry. Try eating at the dinner table before you watch television. You may even find that you'd rather do something else like read the Bible or go exercise!

7. Don't be tricked by "fat-free" food labels.

Some people think that when a cookie package or ice cream container says "fat free" they get a license to pig out. Most of these foods that appear to be healthy are really just loaded with sugar and are a complete waste of calories. I'd rather see you eat a small serving of regular ice cream or cookies than consume huge quantities of the fat-free variety.

8. Don't trick yourself into thinking you're doing things right and not getting results.

Many people who start a program of exercise and nutrition think they're doing the right things when they really aren't, and then they say things like "I can't lose weight," or "I can't gain muscle." This isn't rocket science, people, and the same basic principles of diet and exercise work for nearly everybody! The problem isn't in the nutrition plan or the exercise program, it's usually in ourselves. That's why I encourage all my personal training clients to WRITE DOWN a list of everything they eat for two consecutive days. It's usually a pretty loud wake-up call, and I challenge you to do the same thing. For the next two days, write down every drink, every meal, every piece of candy you consume. Write down the exact serving sizes you take in and the corresponding amount of calories. When you total everything up, I think you'll see that you still need to make some changes!

9. Pack your food for the day.

You must be prepared to resist temptation! This is one of my biggest "pet peeves." I'll write out a meal plan for a client that requires them to pack their lunch and snacks, and the next question I get is, "Can't I just get something healthy at a drive-thru?" NO! Believe me, it's important to take the extra time and discipline required to prepare your meals for the road so you don't find yourself at a fast food place.

10. Learn how to handle restaurants.

If you have to go out to eat, you can still make healthy selections. The first thing to do is skip the alcohol, soft drinks, and coffee and just drink water. If you're out with friends who are all drinking, simply order a sparkling water with lime or lemon. If there are no healthy food choices on the menu, you can politely ask the server if you can order something that isn't on the menu. Just create your own meal that consists of a portion of protein, a portion of carbohydrate, and a portion of fat that suites your taste. For example, you could ask for a grilled chicken breast or a grilled piece of fish with rice and a salad with oil and vinegar. You'll find that most restaurants are happy to accommodate you.

11. If you crave something, have a little, but don't keep it in the house. I'm not trying to create any robots here, I just want you to make better decisions about your eating habits. If you want chocolate you can eat some, but just don't be a glutton. (It's a sin, remember?!) By not keeping chocolate in the house, you'll have to work harder to get it, and you may realize that it's just not worth the effort. And if you do go out to fulfill your craving, just don't over-indulge!

12. At social events, don't sit near a bowl of chips.

Strength is not just the ability to resist temptation, strength is the ability to avoid temptation altogether.

13. If you blow it, don't give up.

Physical fitness is a lifestyle change, not a quick fix. You may experience bumps along the way, but that doesn't mean you have to give it all up. Just pick yourself up, dust yourself off, and start all over again, knowing that every move you make in the right direction is a positive thing. There is no failure. There may be lapses in judgment, but God is always there to give you strength, support, and unending love.

Chapter Eight

The Ten Commandments Of Fitness

"We commit the Golden Rule to memory and forget to commit it to life."
-- Anonymous

Live by these rules and you'll be well on your way to getting your best body — a body filled with energy and vitality that can help you get the most out of life and your relationship with God.

1. Thou shalt perform resistance training in order to increase thy lean muscle.

2. Thou shalt perform cardiovascular exercise at least four times a week, for a minimum of thirty minutes each time, at thy target heart rate.

3. Thou shalt not be obsessed with scale weight and thou shalt learn to understand that even "thin" people can have a high body fat percentage.

4. Thou shalt eat five to six small, portionally correct meals throughout the day in order to increase thy metabolism.

5. Thou shalt consume a minimum of one-half of thy bodyweight in ounces of water on a daily basis.

6. Thou shalt not exercise on an empty stomach to accelerate weight loss.

7. Thou shalt not drastically restrict caloric intake nor deprive thyself of any nutrient, such as carbohydrate, in order to lose weight.

8. Thou shalt make every effort to eat whole, natural foods and limit thy intake of processed powders, bars, and manmade meal replacements.

9. Thou shalt not rely exclusively on fat-burning supplements to accelerate weight loss.

10. Thou shalt understand that God created thee with a unique genetic makeup, and therefore thou shall not covet another person's appearance over thy own.

Chapter Nine

Inspiring Testimony From Christians Living The Lifestyle

"You're never a loser until you quit trying."

-- Mike Ditka

Throughout my career as a personal trainer, model, and motivational speaker, I've met thousands of people striving to live full lives as healthy Christians. I've seen people become active at church after transforming their bodies, because they were no longer embarrassed to be seen in public. I've seen people struggle with physical setbacks and use those experiences to enrich their spiritual lives. I've seen people draw upon their faith to fight for their bodies back after debilitating accidents.

The people I meet in my career inspire me and I've learned so much more than I've been able to teach. Here are just a few stories of people who have found or are looking to find a balance between their physical and spiritual sides. As I see it, these people are "living the lifestyle" and are better Christians as a result.

Chapter Ten

Fit for Marriage

The Story of Fred and Stephanie Morales

"We were no longer able to use the normal excuses,
such as 'no time to work out' or 'I'm too tired.'"

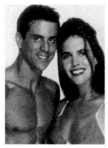

Fred and Stephanie had been married for six years when they decided to do something about their bodies. While they were determined to achieve physical results, they had no idea that working together to get in shape would deepen the sacrament they shared together.

"On the surface, our life seemed good," says Fred. "Our marriage was working, we had two beautiful children, and we lived in sunny Southern California!

"We knew, however, that something was missing. Looking back, it's easy to see that being fat put a cloud over our lives. But at the time, we didn't even realize that we were deliberately staying away from 'embarrassing' situations like going to the beach with the kids.

"On a typical day, I'd work, pick up some fast food and beer on the way home, and fall asleep in front of the TV. Stephanie had just had our second child and complained about her appearance. I looked in the mirror myself, and for the first time I noticed the 30 pounds I had gained since college.

"Stephanie and I both decided to make a change. I went to the grocery store and decided to buy a fitness magazine. That month, Muscle & Fitness featured a cover model with a more natural, fit, and healthy look. It was Clark Bartram.

"I bought the magazine and started to flip through the pages. I came to an ad for a physique transformation contest that offered money, cars, and vacations to people who could get in great shape in 12 weeks. That was the motivation we needed, so Stephanie and I joined the contest.

"Like the saying goes, God works in mysterious ways, and we actually met Clark Bartram through a mutual friend. Clark mapped out a plan for us that included exercise, nutrition, and supplements, and he helped us keep our commitment to complete the challenge.

"The hardest part was the first couple of weeks, because our habits had to change. We were no longer able to use the normal excuses, such as 'no time to work out' or 'I'm too tired.'

"Going through this difficult time actually brought Stephanie and I closer together. For the first time in quite awhile, we were really communicating. We helped each other reach our goals, we encouraged each other, and we created a healthy new life pattern that involved the whole family.

"For example, we began eating meals together at the dinner table, which brought us closer to our two boys. This simple change gave us quality time as a family, and Stephanie and I were able to get more involved in our children's lives.

"It wasn't long before we noticed our bodies responding to Clark's program, too, and that motivated us to keep pursuing our fitness goals and share our experiences with others. Our whole attitude about life changed for the better. Going to Church on Sundays was now fun because we had a deeper connection as a married couple. Going to the beach was no longer embarrassing, and we were finally free to share in the sense of fun and wonder that came so naturally to our kids.

"Ultimately, Stephanie and I won second place in the physique transformation contest, and we knew that we couldn't have done it without each other. While we're tremendously proud of our achievement, we now realize that fitness is a lifelong pursuit, not just something you do to win a prize. For us, the real prize has been the realization that, as a committed couple sharing the sacrament of marriage, we are much stronger than two individuals. We know that together, we can do anything, and that has made us better spouses, as well as better parents.

"I can honestly say that the only downside to the whole experience has been Stephanie's newfound love for clothes shopping!"

Chapter Eleven

Resurrection

The Story of James DeMelo

"Someone once told me that the only thing that stands between a man and what he wants from life is the will to try and the faith to believe it is possible."

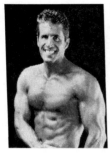

On April 24, 1998, James DeMelo was in a critical accident. A semi-truck hit his car, and the impact literally left him dead at the scene. There was a paramedic on the corner, and when he rushed to the car and checked James's vitals, he couldn't feel a pulse. But he began CPR and James's heart began to beat again. Through the grace of God his life was saved, but he had broken his neck in two places, his back was broken in four places, his shoulder blade and a couple of ribs were broken, and he suffered various other injuries.

"I wore a halo brace on my head for three months so the neck vertebrae could heal," explains James. "But even after that I had a long way to go in the recovery process. Significant nerve damage remained, and a large portion of my muscle mass had atrophied. I had so much to overcome, and I wasn't sure I could do it.

"But I had to try. Someone once told me that the only thing that stands between a man and what he wants from life is the will to try and the faith to believe it is possible. At first it was difficult, but I forced myself to go to the gym twice a day. Within the first two weeks I had increased my strength and stamina, and my mobility had greatly improved. I began to see that it was possible to regain my quality of life.

"After three months of consistent workouts, a healthy diet, and nutritional supplements, I lost 16 pounds of fat and regained 11 pounds of lean muscle mass. Eight weeks into the program, I felt so good that I was able to minister for a week in Ghana, West Africa. When I started, I couldn't do 15 minutes of cardio or play with my daughter for more than a few minutes at a time. I couldn't lift heavy things or do yard work. I didn't know if any of these things would ever be possible again. Now I can say to anyone who's been injured — it is possible to recover, it is possible to regain, and it is possible to reclaim your life.

"My life has been devoted to helping people spiritually, but now I know that I can encourage people physically as well. I'm an example of what can be achieved with dedication, hard work, and God's help. Already, I've been able to motivate those in the gym who watched my metamorphosis. I truly believe that there's opportunity in the middle of every difficulty, and that the fullness or emptiness of life is measured by the extent to which we feel we have an impact on others. That's why I'll keep reaching out, however I can, even if it's just being able to say, 'Hey, I did it — so can you.'

"I saw my rehab doctor a year after my accident, and he couldn't believe the progress I had made. But for me, it wasn't just the physical changes that have made a difference in my life. While those things are important, and I'm happy that I can run and play with my little girls and teach them soccer and softball, the real peace of mind comes from knowing that my faith can help me overcome any obstacle life throws at me.

"Throughout my life, I've found that when you help others reach their dreams, you usually reach yours in the process. So I tell people, 'You can change your life! Don't focus on what you are, but on what you can become.'"

Chapter Twelve

Keeping The Faith

The Story of Julia Zaher

"I'll do anything to lose weight — except eat right and exercise!"

My friend Julia has been struggling to get her weight down. She tends to start into things with a little too much enthusiasm, and then she'll just get completely sidetracked. I think a lot of people share this pattern, but Julia's learning from her experiences and she's smart enough to keep a sense of humor about the whole thing. She knows that her goals are attainable, and she trusts that God will help her find the right time to make them happen.

"I'll do anything to lose weight," Julia says. "Except eat right and exercise! That's too basic. Give me pills, powders, homeopathic remedies, or the latest diet that promises to help me lose 20 pounds in two weeks. But when I look back on the years when I've lost weight, put on muscle, and felt great, none of those get-thin-quick schemes could take the credit. I turn to those things in a panic when I gain weight. We all want the quick fix. The only thing I've ever found that got the weight off and kept it off is a lifestyle of healthy eating and daily exercise.

"Two years ago, I was well over 200 pounds and about a size 18. I hated shopping and seldom took a good look at myself in the mirror. Then I decided to participate in a body transformation contest. A friend took my picture in a two-piece bathing suit and I was truly horrified by the much-needed reality check. I got busy. I spent hours and hours in the gym, hired a personal trainer, took supplements, and even underwent hypnosis to help change my negative mental images. I did experience a fairly dramatic transformation. I lost 20 pounds on the scale, but through body fat analysis I knew I'd lost even more fat while gaining muscle.

"Someone at the gym asked where this tremendous motivation to change had come from. He was surprised to hear me say it came out of my prayer times. For many months, the Lord had very tenderly been calling me to take better care of my body. The words I heard in my heart were, "I need you to lose weight and get in shape. It's preparation for what lies ahead." So I set out to lose the weight out of obedience to

God and a desire to be healthier and happier. I was on my way to a permanent life as a thin person.

"Fast forward two years later. I've regained the 20 pounds. I still have some of the muscle I gained from my diligent, although excessive workouts. But somewhere along the line, going to the gym ceased to be a priority. Eating right gave way to eating whatever I wanted. And here I am starting all over again.

"What's really pathetic is that I have friends like fitness model Clark Bartram who have been incredibly encouraging. My job as a radio producer allowed me to spend an entire day last year with seven-time Mr. Olympia, Lee Haney, another tremendous Christian man and fitness expert. And yet even with God orchestrating all of these wonderful connections, left on my own at home I reverted to my old habits in a little more than a year after tasting success. What was my problem?

"My problem is my priorities. When eating regular, balanced meals becomes an irregular practice, when going to the gym becomes an optional activity in the day, I'm in trouble. I finally confessed my relapse to Clark and then he did what all loving friends do — he asked me to write about it in his book. Thanks for this exercise in humility, Clark!

"I've seen what's happened when people follow Clark's advice on eating right and training smart. They get results. Clark even warned me about some of the things I was doing wrong in my initial fitness quest. I was taking advice from too many people, jumping from program to program. I was spending too much time in the gym, not realizing that weight training is not an endurance sport. It's about brief, but focused and intense effort.

"So I've picked up Clark's beginning weight training program and I'm starting again. Being overweight and out of shape for life is not an option. I still believe God has a plan, and that plan requires me to have the stamina to do whatever He asks of me.

"The Bible tells us to love the Lord with all our hearts, and to love our neighbor as ourselves. Taking good care of my body is one way I love myself. It allows me to be more loving to others. God has also taught me about the unconditional nature of true love. Whether we are fat or thin, God loves us. I appreciate the fact that Clark didn't get on my case when he heard that I gained the weight back. Instead, he lovingly encouraged me to get off the couch and get to the gym. He knows the kind of person I am on the inside and wants to see that reflected on the outside.

"Living a committed Christian life means going against the grain of our culture. Eating right and working out regularly are also counter-cultural. Wouldn't it be great if people thought of Christians as being the healthiest, most balanced people they know? That's what I'm aiming for and I'll keep disciplining my mind, my body, and my spirit to that end."

Chapter Thirteen

Faith and Fitness — Life's Non-Negotiables

The Story of Bill Arnold

"Try your gimmicks if you must, but I promise you the truth is in the basics. Make it fun. Be creative. Challenge yourself, but also cut yourself some slack."

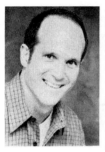

My buddy Bill is one of the funniest guys I've ever met. He's on the road all the time, but he's managed to make his health and his faith the two top priorities in his life. Here's his story and advice in his own words: "I think Allen Konigsberg said, '90 percent of life is just showing up.'

That's pretty simple! Invite discipline in (show up at the gym and actually work out) and watch it act like your best friend. Discipline gets a bad rap, but it's really our pal! Discipline liberates us. If you have the discipline to train hard, you have the freedom to enjoy a strong body. If you have the discipline to eat well, the energy you get gives you the freedom to live life to the fullest!

"In my business as an actor and magician, I need all the energy and strength I can get to grind out seven shows a week doing physically demanding comedy.

"But I have a ton of excuses not to stay disciplined. (Like, it's Tuesday.) Last year I was on the road for 26 weeks. It can be stressful being displaced from the comforts of home, church, family, and friends. Finding yourself hungry in an airport, lost in a city trying to find a gym, or just flat out lonely, can eat away at your will power to stay focused on the goals you've set for yourself.

"I have little daily goals I call "non-negotiables." Unless it's a rest day or a predetermined time off for recovery, getting in a workout for the last 26 years has been a non-negotiable. I don't make excuses, I do it. It's a lot like prayer and my desire to be connected to Jesus, my source of strength. My prayer life is another non-negotiable.

"I encourage you to develop your own non-negotiables. Maybe one is to tell your spouse every day that "I choose you and I love you." Maybe another is like mine — to work out and pray every day. Maybe you'll have a non-negotiable against gossip or pettiness, or maybe you'll have a non-negotiable to be your own best friend. Building these disciplines and sticking to them will be a huge boost in your life. Remember, discipline's your pal!

The first thing you need to do is get good information. When it comes to fitness, Clark has helped me gain perspective and face reality! There are no short cuts, and there's no fooling anybody (tough words for a magician to hear). Hard work plus diet and exercise is the only route to a better body.

Try your gimmicks if you must, but I promise you the truth is in the basics.

Make it fun. Be creative. Challenge yourself, but also cut yourself some slack. Don't obsess about the little things you don't like about your physique (like no quad development, phantom calves, minimal size with little definition in your back, pecs, and shoulders). So you haven't put a millimeter on your arms in the last ten years — anybody can have an off decade! Not everybody can look like Clark, but you can put your mind to it and (without sounding too sappy) be the best you can be. And that's a thrill!

At 44, it's still fun when someone guesses my age to be only 43 and a half! I love the challenge of changing my physique through diet and exercise.

It's a huge battle to effect a change. Your body fights to stay where it's at. So be smart about your nutrition, training, and rest. Stack the deck in your favor! Be encouraged. Train for a lifetime, don't set it up as a quick fix. You might become disillusioned and write if off as something you can't succeed at. When you're traveling, be innovative! Some of the best little exercises I've discovered or invented have come as a result of having limited equipment. Don't walk into a poorly equipped hotel gym and get discouraged. Get inventive! You'll have to if your goal is non-negotiable!

Clark has inspired me with his encouragement, and by the knowledge that he shares through his articles, TV shows, videos, and books. He's easy to admire because of his no nonsense approach that says with the right tools and the right attitude you will be a success.

Thanks Clark, for leading by example, being humble about what God has blessed you with, and providing the most readable stuff on the fitness market.

Oh, by the way, Allen Konigsberg is better known as Woody Allen. I'm a magician — I had to try to fool you at least once!

Chapter Fourteen

Doing It For The Right Reasons

The Story of Anita Bartram

"Just because I'm married to the guy who wrote this book doesn't mean that keeping fit is any easier for me. In fact, it can be even harder sometimes."

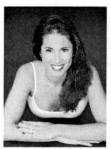

You get to pick up my book whenever you want to, but my beautiful wife Anita has to live with me all the time! My 'round-the-clock involvement in the fitness industry has created some extra pressures for the people who are closest to me, and they've had to work a little harder to figure out why it's really good for them to exercise and eat right. But I'll let Anita tell you all about it herself:

"Just because I'm married to the guy who wrote this book doesn't mean that keeping fit is any easier for me. In fact, it can be even harder sometimes.

"Some of the people Clark runs into in his line of work can be pretty superficial, and for some reason they hold me to a higher standard. They have this preconceived notion that I must be this perfect, flawless creature, and I often find myself thinking that I'm supposed to live up to their false standards.

"And then there are all the women Clark works with. I admit I have a hard time with that sometimes. Not because I don't trust Clark, but because I tend to compare myself to the "perfect" images these girls convey in their photographs. That can be a lot of pressure!

"To top it all off, I seem to be a living example of the scripture that says familiarity breeds contempt. I know Clark's an expert who can get anyone in the best shape possible — I've seen it happen countless times with his clients and fans who tell him how he's been an inspiration to them. But I often find myself not wanting advice from him. I guess I just take it too personally. Even if I ask him a question and he innocently says something like 'maybe those chips aren't such a great idea,' I hear 'you're fat and out of shape!'

"Clark doesn't put any pressure on me, but I sure put pressure on myself! It's something I've had to work through, and as challenging as it's been it's helped me grow. I'm not out of shape, but I could do better. I may indulge in a snack from time to time (by the way, so does Clark, but don't tell him I told you that!) but I try not to overdo it. And let me tell you, when you're surrounded by people who are paid to stay super-fit all the time, you tend to get a little self-conscious no matter how good a shape you're in!

"For me, fitness isn't a profession, but it's important in my life. When I stop comparing myself to others, when I keep things in the right perspective, I find great pleasure and joy in exercise and good nutrition. I exercise and eat right because it feels good, and also because I want to set a good example for my children. My kids love to exercise because they see how much fun Clark and I have being active, and they love to pray and go to Church because they see that we take our spiritual side very seriously, too.

"The two things go hand in hand, and I've even noticed that I exercise more when I pray more. I tend to withdraw and not do much of anything when I'm not purposefully investing time in prayer, and I benefit more in every aspect of my life when I consistently pray and ask God to help me deal with my insecurities.

"I love being married to Clark, and our relationship has stood the test of time because it has many dimensions — physical as well as spiritual. I may get frustrated or intimidated by his profession sometimes, but I know that's an illusion that isn't real. Maybe you've had the same pressures from images you've seen on TV or in magazines. Believe me, all those people aren't perfect (I've met a lot of them and they don't even pretend to be!) and if you can relax, try not be so hard on yourself, and get in shape for the right reasons for you, I think your fitness endeavors will be a lot more fun and a lot easier, too."

Chapter Fifteen

A Balanced Workout

"Everything in life seemed to be a struggle, both physically and mentally"

by John Riccio

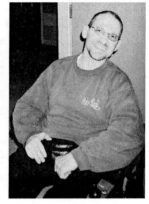

Life is a journey filled with many different experiences. Walking on this road we are constantly learning, growing, changing and maturing in the hope that each day will better than the next. I hope and pray that by sharing what I have gone through and learned this will bless you in a positive way.

I was born with a birth defect called Cerebral Palsy. Only three pounds at birth, I spent the first two months of my life in an incubator. The doctors would tell my mother she should get rid of me because I won't live long anyway. Everything in life seemed to be a struggle both physically and emotionally. The simplest tasks that most people take for granted took hours for me to complete. People would stare or children would laugh. I felt as though I was not of any value. At this point you are probably asking yourself where is the blessing in this?

I was only able to watch television as a child and my dream was to be healthy and strong. One day I saw a guy named Jack LaLanne on the T.V. and I knew that is what I wanted in life. The burning desire I had didn't begin take shape until fifteen years from the time I saw Jack LaLanne on television. The first I went to the gym I had to be carried down the stairs to the weight room. Talk about humble beginning. Time went by and I was faithfully pursuing my dream. From age 19 to 26 I had accomplished all I set out to do. I had management positions in two health clubs. Competed in bodybuilding, placing in every show against able bodied individuals. I was also on local television and in two bodybuilding magazines for my efforts. In 1993, while getting ready to compete in a big bodybuilding contest, I felt a great deal of pain in my feet. Knowing something was wrong I went to the hospital. Realizing I needed an operation, meant I would be unable to compete . Two years of training down the drain with nothing to show for it. The show was only four weeks away and there I was at 5 % body fat hoping to qualify for the NPC Nationals. The operation took a toll on body. My heart rate was down to 8 to 10 beats per minute. I slipped into a coma for three days. I really needed to look at my life in a different way. Everything I did for the last 10 years was geared toward my physique. I missed out on the simple joy of realizing each day is a precious gift. Ten years have passed since then. Through God's grace and patience He has shown me that we were never put here to compete with one another but to help complete one another. The greatest desire I have now is to encourage and motivate others in a kind and loving manner, spiritually, mentally or physically. Balance is the key to walking as it is in life. Being the best is ok as long as it doesn't bring out the worst. I continue to learn to be humble, gentle, meek and lowly not hard, harsh, sharp or pressing. One of life's greatest joys is being at peace no matter what the circumstances are around you so you can fully enjoy the walk of life. Even if you walk it with crutches.

Chapter Sixteen

Afterword

"Never, never, never give up."

-- Winston Churchill

Now what? Now that you're armed with all of this useful information, what will you do with it? We all know the scripture in the Bible, "zeal without knowledge is useless" (Proverbs 19:2). I guess that could be reversed to say, "knowledge without zeal is useless," too.
Another scripture (2 Peter 5-8) may motivate you to put your newfound fitness knowledge into action:
"...make every effort to supplement your faith with goodness, goodness with knowledge, knowledge with self-control, self-control with endurance, endurance with Godliness, Godliness with brotherly affection, and brotherly affection with love. For if these qualities are yours and are increasing, they will keep you from being useless or unfruitful in the knowledge of our Lord Jesus Christ."
You might be wondering how this scripture directly relates to your fitness regimen. Simply think of your health, exercise program, and good nutrition as examples of the "goodness" spoken of in the passage as a supplement to your faith, and everything expands from there. You might even consider making this scripture your daily prayer or meditation in regards to your fitness program. If you do, I'll bet you'll achieve tremendous results!

Simple Things You Can Do To Get Started Now
1. Begin to take deeper breaths, this will allow the oxygen to flow more readily through your body.
2. Put down the coffee or soda and pick up some water.
3. Stand up right now and move. Get the blood moving through your body.
4. Make a commitment to exercise by finding an accountability partner, just as you should in your spiritual life.
5. Write down everything you eat and drink for the next two days. This will help you understand exactly what is going into your body. I'll say it again — write it down!

6. Once you have your list, make subtle changes in your eating habits. If you're eating too much candy for example, cut the amount in half.
7. Take a photo of yourself and place it on your refrigerator for motivation. Like you saw in Julia's testimony, the "wake-up call" of her photo propelled her to make a lifelong decision to live healthier.
8. Write down your affirmations.
9. Begin to say your affirmations aloud daily, three times a day or whenever you feel like giving up or giving in.
10. Pray about the balance God would have you keep throughout this wonderful, life-changing experience.

As I look back over my life and reflect on the blessings that God has given and continues to give me, I feel a sense of awe as I remember the person I once was. The guy who was thinking only of himself, who treated those he cared about with less respect than they deserved, and who didn't have time for God in his life. That same person is now blossoming into more of what God would expect of His creation.

I grow and learn each day and continue to make mistakes along the way, but I'll never let that stop me in my pursuit of being all God wants me to be and has predestined for me. A friend of mine often says, "I may not be where I wanna be, but thank God I'm not where I used to be!"

Just think, if I wasn't challenged by that skinny young Christian man in 1988 and continued to procrastinate about my eternal fate, I may have continued to have that sense that something was wrong inside despite outward appearances. I may have lost the woman who has stood by me all the way, and with whom I share the blessings of two wonderful children. Man, am I glad that I accepted that challenge! If I hadn't, I would have missed out on the spiritual richness that God had already prepared for me.

My friends, it's now my turn to challenge you! Will you be all that you can be, physically AND spiritually? Or will you live a life that's out of balance and less than God wants for you? Your body is a blessing from God, and it's time to stop abusing this precious gift.

As in salvation, no one can make the decision for you and you are left with the results of your choice. But if you've read this far, I'm confident that you'll make the right move. As the Bible says (Deuteronomy 30:19) **"...I set before you life and death, blessing and curses. Now choose life so that you and your children may live."**

Acknowledgements

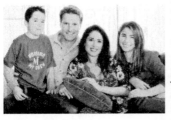

My deepest gratitude goes to **Anita, Taylor,** and **Mitch.** The three of you are my constant source of inspiration and happiness.

Jason Ellis, thank you for your continual support and photographic genius — on to the next project, my friend!

Bill Arnold, you are a true friend. I appreciate all you've done for me, and for helping make this book a reality. Now you can finally get in shape!

William Smith, CEO/President of INTRAFITT Corp., thanks for lending your time and expertise on nutrition to help make this project first-rate. I know you have many things on your plate — no pun intended!

Nick at Escondido Workout, thanks for allowing me to shoot in your great gym.

Ed Sweet, you make me sound great — what a talent you have.

Pastor Daniel, you are a shining example of a Godly man. Thanks for being a true friend.

James DeMelo, thanks for expecting the most out of me, both physically and spiritually. You've been a great mentor.

Mom, Dad, Michelle, Rocco, and **Jason** — each of you are special to me.

Roger and everyone at Hoist, thanks for helping me out all the time.

Ralph DeHaan, you are a great friend. Thanks for supporting me with your photographic talents.

David Sparks, thanks for your unselfish attitude and willingness to use your God given artistic talent to design my book. I am truly grateful and wish you much success in all of your many projects.

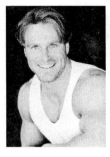 Clark Bartram has earned his reputation as "America's Most Trusted Fitness Personality." In everything he does, Clark puts forth 100% in the hopes that he can benefit men and women who care enough about themselves and the people they love to do what it takes to "Live the Lifestyle."

As a professional fitness model, Clark has appeared on the cover of countless magazines, including Muscle & Fitness and Natural Bodybuilding.

As a personal trainer, Clark has helped hundreds of men and women transform their bodies and their lives. Clark has inspired millions of television viewers as the co-host of Kiana's Flex Appeal on ESPN, and currently shares his wealth of knowledge on exercise and nutrition as the host of American Health & Fitness, broadcast internationally.

Clark regularly contributes articles to national fitness magazines like Ironman and Muscle Media, and is also the author of the how-to guide, You Too Can Be A Fitness Model.

He recently introduced the Clark Bartram Nutrition for Fitness supplement line and describes himself as an evangelist for honest nutrition at an excellent value.

As a Christian, Clark is actively involved with the Prison Fellowship/Operation Starting Line as a national artist doing in-prison evangelism. He has worked with the Billy Graham Evangelistic Association as an emcee for the Franklin Graham Crusades, and, through the Men's Ministry at his own church, gives motivational speeches at school and community events.

In addition to his full-time fitness career and his ministry, Clark is a devoted husband and father.

For more information about Clark Bartram, visit his Web site at **www.clarkbartram.com.**

Ten Good Reasons To Drink Water

1. Life itself can't exist without water. Humans can go for weeks with out food, but only 3 days without water.

2. About 70% of your body is water. Water makes up nearly 85 percent of your brain, 80 percent of your blood, and 70 percent of your lean muscle. We must constantly add fresh water to our bodies to keep them properly hydrated.

3. Water plays a vital role in nearly every bodily function. Water is essential for digestion, nutrient absorption, chemical reactions, circulation, waste elimination, and temperature regulation.

4. Lack of water is the #1 trigger of daytime fatigue. When your body is well hydrated, your blood oxygen levels increase and you have more energy. Dehydration can lead to decreased motor skills, concentration and memory retention.

5. When you're dehydrated, you tend to eat more. Water suppresses the appetite naturally and helps the body metabolize stored fat. Recent studies indicate that nearly 40% of the American population suffers daily from a false sense of hunger due to moderate levels of dehydration. Other research has shown that even mild dehydration may slow the metabolic rate by as much as 3-5%.

6. Water can be a miracle cure for headaches, joint pain, and other ailments. Dehydration can lead to increased back and joint pain in up to 80% of the people suffering from these symptoms.

7. Consistent lack of water can lead to Chronic Cellular Dehydration. This condition weakens the body's immune system and leads to chemical, nutritional, and pH imbalances that can cause a host of diseases.

8. Dehydration can occur year-round. Winter dryness can dehydrate the body even quicker than summer heat.

9. It's difficult for the body to get water from any other source. Soft drinks, coffee, tea, and alcohol actually steal tremendous amounts of water from the body.

10. Dehydration can increase your risk of colon, breast, and bladder cancer.

50 Prayers and Meditations...

....And Affirmations To Help You Get Fit And Live A Healthier, Happier Life

1. Dear Heavenly Father, I thank you for my body and my ability to move, breathe, and function efficiently. I choose not to take my body for granted, and I decide today to pay more attention to drinking water, eating healthy, exercising, and focusing on the positive.

2. I have the opportunity today to start fresh and begin to live a healthier lifestyle. I choose to see myself in a new, more positive light. I thank you, God, for new beginnings.

3. I ask for the strength to deal with my weaknesses. I ask for focus to follow through with commitments. I ask for wisdom to make the right decisions. I ask for patience in my relationships. And I ask for humility to keep me balanced as my body begins to change and respond to my fitness regimen.

4. Dear God, I ask that you give me a new understanding of what happens when I abuse my body with drugs and alcohol. Let me see my current behavior for what it really is and open my eyes to a better way of living.

5. Lord, please give me the desire to exercise and eat right consistently, and don't allow me to get depressed or put unnecessary pressure on myself when I fall short. I realize I am not perfect-no one is. I ask for the ability to get up, shake off the dust, and start fresh without the guilt of feeling like a loser.

6. Please don't let me look upon anyone else with coveting eyes. I realize that I am a unique Creation, and that there is nobody else like me. I understand that there are some people I will never look like, and I choose today not to compare myself to others in an unhealthy way.

7. Please go with me as I walk into the gym and protect my eyes and mind from lusting over anybody I may be attracted to. I desire to have an effective and meaningful workout, and I decide not to allow my pursuit of a healthier body to be hindered by a wandering eye or lustful mind. I also choose not to engage in any meaningless conversations in the gym that will distract me from my goals.

8. Please keep me safe in the gym and during my workout.

9. Please allow me to see the results of my efforts to improve my body and my health-even small ones-so that I may stay motivated to achieve my goals. I want results from my program and would love to see some tangible signs to keep me on track, such as weight loss, compliments from people, and increased energy.

10. As I progress in my discipline and begin to see solid results, please allow me to be an encouragement to someone else that may be struggling with their health or their body. I desire not only to get in shape for myself, but also to be an encouragement to others.

11. I choose today to be a shining example of healthy choices to my children, friends, spouse, co-workers, and anyone else who is closely connected to me in life. I realize that there is much more to being in shape and living a healthy lifestyle than mere appearances.

12. Heavenly Father, let me pursue a healthy lifestyle for all the right reasons. I understand that I want to look better, but there are other, more important, reasons to get in shape, such as the possibility of a longer life, the chance to be a good example to others, the capacity to be more productive, and the ability to serve You better.

13. Please prevent my new body from becoming a point of contention between my spouse and me. I ask that he or she be understanding, supportive, and encouraging. I also ask for his or her assistance in keeping me accountable and on track toward my goals. I also ask that any compliments I may receive from the opposite sex will not cause problems in my marriage. Please give me the ability and strength to have open communication with my spouse so no wedge is placed between us.

14. Dear God, I ask for a humble spirit when I begin to get results from my fitness program. I realize that increased confidence can be often misinterpreted as arrogance. Please don't let me be proud, haughty, conceited, or a show off with my new body.

15. Heavenly Father, be with me every day, especially when I am weak and want to cheat. As I drive past my favorite fast food restaurant, please give me the strength to avoid the drive-thru lane. When I am grocery shopping, please help me make healthy choices and not be fooled by false claims and deceitful advertisements.

16. Dear Lord, please let me see my value as a person first and don't allow me to think that if I become more fit I will have more value. I understand that appearances don't measure value-character does. I know that I am already a special person, and that You and many people in my life love me exactly how I am today.

17. Please work on me from the inside out. For every minute I devote to my physical body, let me have the strength and courage to devote at least that amount to my spiritual education, prayer, and devotional time.

18. My Lord, give me the strength to overcome any weakness, whether it be emotional, physical, spiritual, mental, or financial. I know there are many things in life that cause confusion and frustration, but I refuse to give them too much significance, especially when it comes to interfering with my workouts.

19. Please don't allow my past failures plague my mind and deceive me into thinking I can't achieve my fitness goals. I understand that failures and mistakes are inevitable, and that the true measure of a person lies in how he or she moves on from them. I ask today for the ability to overcome my past and see progress as I set out to improve my present and future. Don't allow my mind to play tricks on me when things get difficult. I know that what I am doing will be rewarded with results, so please give me the reassurance I need in order to push through the tough days, hours, minutes, and moments. I can reach my goals with Your help, Heavenly Father, so please be with me every step of the way and be that voice in my head that whispers, "You can do it-don't stop"!

20. Allow my pursuit of fitness to be a fun experience, and please don't let me see exercise as a burden. I choose to go forward with a "can-do" attitude and enjoy every challenge and achievement.

21. I ask you Father, to put the right person of the same gender in my life to motivate me, encourage me, inspire me, and hold me accountable to my commitment to achieve better health and fitness. I choose to allow myself the luxury of understanding that I can't do this alone and I am willing and asking for guidance and direction. I understand that having an "accountability partner" will increase my chances of success.

22. I ask that my quest for fitness doesn't become an obsession for me like it has in the past. Fitness is important to me, but it is not the only thing that's important in my life. Dear God, please let me understand how to place my fitness goals in the bigger picture of my life.

23. I ask that my pursuit of a healthy lifestyle will draw my family closer together. Heavenly Father, make me a positive example for my spouse and children of what good food and exercise choices can do for someone.

24. Please allow me to love myself as I currently am. I am important and valuable regardless of my weight, size, or physical shortcomings.

25. I ask that you renew my mind and take away my pattern of self-abuse. Negative self-talk-which wrongfully causes me to believe things like "I'm fat," "I'm ugly," or "I'm useless"-no longer belongs in my life. I also ask that you help me

stop me from eating myself into depression, or from the vicious cycle of binging and purging. Take all unhealthy eating habits away from me completely and give me the strength to resist food temptations.

26. Lord, please give me wisdom and guidance when it comes to spending my hard earned money on supplements, gym memberships, trainers, and other items that can easily be misrepresented. I ask for discernment when it comes to crafty advertisements pitching false claims. And please do not let me be tricked into thinking there is a miracle pill or potion. I understand that a fitness lifestyle takes consistent effort and discipline. I ask that you give me that today.

27. Please help me focus on the basics. I understand that there is no quick fix or easy way of developing healthy lifestyle patterns. I am engaging myself in a process of basic principles that will eventually lead me to a strong, energetic, and physically fit body. I need help, so I am calling out today and asking that you guide me every step of the way.

28. I have so much to be thankful for. I choose today to see my life as a blessing, not a curse. I choose to look at myself as a beautiful, productive, energetic person who is capable of anything I set out to do. I ask for a new perspective on life and especially on how I see things in my mind's eye. I choose not to focus on unimportant, meaningless things that cause me stress. I will be a positive, caring, considerate person and realize how good I really do have it.

29. Please help me wake up early in the morning. I choose not to sleep my life away. I have decided to invest that extra time in the morning to a health and fitness regimen. I desire to be a joyful person in the morning and to use that time productively.

30. Please give me grace when it comes to dealing with my children and their eating habits. Don't allow me to speak anything that would adversely affect their lives or cause them to have negative self-images. I desire to be a positive influence both in my words and actions.

31. I choose to forgive anyone who may have said, or will in the future say something hurtful or negative about my appearance or about my efforts to pursue a healthy lifestyle. I will no longer allow my self-image to be dictated by others.

32. I choose today to let go of bitterness. Bitterness can cause unnecessary stress, anger, and self-abuse, and I have no room in my new life for those negative elements. Nothing that takes away from my emotional or physical well-being is worth my time or energy.

33. I choose to have fun with my fitness program and not stress or obsess over minor details. I will maintain a healthy and positive attitude about my fitness regimen.

34. I feel great, I look great, and I am loved!

35. I choose today to enter into my fitness program with a positive, focused, and determined mindset. I will have success and I will have a great workout today.

36. I will do today what is necessary to become what I want to be tomorrow.

37. I realize that the secret of health-in both mind and body-is not to fret about the past, worry about the future, or anticipate troubles, but to live in the present moment wisely and earnestly.

38. I choose today to believe in myself and have faith in my abilities. I will be successful if I have a humble and reasonable confidence in myself.

39. I realize that my mental and physical condition is a direct reflection of my current state of mind. I choose today to change the way I think about myself.

40. I understand that the first step in getting what I want out of life is deciding what I want specifically and writing it down.

41. Success in life is peace of mind, which comes from the knowledge that I am doing my best to become the best I can be.

42. I know the secret to productive goal setting is to establish clearly defined goals. I will write down and focus on my goals several times a day as if I have already achieved them, with words, pictures, and emotions. Example: "I feel great in my size 6 jeans!"

43. I realize the importance of preparation. I will be prepared to face temptation. I will have my clothes ready for the gym on my scheduled days and I will not make excuses. I realize that I will eventually drive past my favorite fast food restaurant, but I will not stop.

44. I understand that time passes by with each excuse. I choose today to stop wasting time and instead invest in my health and fitness program. I do this to make the most of each moment in my life.

45. I understand that I will have to make certain sacrifices in order to achieve the healthy and fit body I desire. I also realize that these sacrifices are well worth the

end result. I am changing day by day and choose today to make the right choices.

46. I realize that it is not what I am that holds me back; it is who I think I am. I choose today to have a positive self-image and know that I am capable of achieving my goals.

47. I choose to do something every day that will bring me one step closer to my goal of a healthier body.

48. I choose not to wait any longer to start living healthier, because I realize that the time will never be 'just right'. I am starting today, and I will work with the tools I have to become healthier by exercising and eating right.

49. I realize that being "motivated" is what gets me started, but it is the habit I create that will keep me consistently achieving goals. I am developing positive "lifestyle" habits that will bring me long-term success.

50. I am a child of God, created in His image. He has given me everything I need to succeed in all areas of my life. I choose today to reflect upon His sovereign power and love for me. I love myself, and I know that I am capable of greatness.

I Am A Winner!